The Puzzling Child: From Recognition to Treatment

The *Journal of Children in Contemporary Society* series:

- *Young Children in a Computerized Environment*
- *Primary Prevention for Children & Families*
- *The Puzzling Child: From Recognition to Treatment*
- *Children of Exceptional Parents*
- *Childhood Depression*

The Puzzling Child: From Recognition to Treatment

Edited by
Mary Frank, MS in Education

Journal of Children in Contemporary Society
Volume 14, Number 4

The Haworth Press
New York

The Haworth Press, Inc., 28 East 22 Street, New York, NY 10010.

Library of Congress Cataloging in Publication Data
Main entry under title:

The Puzzling child.

(Journal of children in contemporary society ; v. 14, no.4)
Includes bibliographical references.
1. Child psychopathology—Diagnosis. 2. Mental health care teams. I. Frank, Mary (Mary Isabelle) II. Series.

RJ503.5.P88 1982	618.92'89075	82-11692

ISBN 0-86656-119-6

The Puzzling Child: From Recognition to Treatment

Journal of Children in Contemporary Society
Volume 14, Number 4

Contents

The Puzzling Child: From Recognition to Treatment

INTRODUCTION

All too frequently, professionals who are providing direct services to young children are heard to say: "We know this child has a problem, but we don't know what it is." This child is the "Puzzling Child," the child who cannot sit quietly for more than a few seconds, the electively mute child who refuses to talk outside the home, the child who does not participate in cooperative play, the child who cannot listen and remember a sequence of spoken information, or the child with a temperament that is classified as slow-to-warm-up and is frequently equated by teachers as being a child with low intellectual capabilities. In fact, the latter is not always true.

Many of these children will require further assessment and treatment. The professionals, with appropriate assessment instruments, the knowledge required to interpret and identify the assessed behavior, and the ability to make a diagnosis, can prescribe a treatment plan. The process may be a simple one or, depending on the complexities of the behavior, may necessitate repeating parts of the process at different times, but using different instruments, different approaches to interpretation, and developing different treatment goals. Because of the multiple dimensions of this process, the articles in this issue address themselves to the practical application of informal assessment, the absence of developmental milestones which are part of the puzzling child's behavior as well as some of the professional and societal issues which impinge on the process "From Recognition to Treatment." The articles, comprehensive in nature and yet practical and applicable in contents, will be of value to those who are in training in the human services and to those who have day-to-day contact with the "puzzling child" in the fields of education, social services, psychology, and pediatric medicine.

Initially, the most accessible assessment method is the observation process. Frequently, this process is of more value than other standardized measures as the child can be observed in his or her natural setting and over a longer period of time. The formalized process is constrained by unnatural settings, unfamiliar people, and limited time. As valuable as the observation process is, and as simple as it sounds, observation principles (Foley) and observation techniques (Cartwright) underline the success of this process. Other informal instruments, the questionnaire (Fox) and the informal interview (Liden and alluded to by Curry), are means of assessment too, but are less accessible to on-line professionals. Ideally, an assessment which follows a multidisciplinary model is more comprehensive as it lends validity and clarity to the interpretation process (Liden).

Interpreting assessments is the real crux, and often the most difficult task, as no behavior is, generally, caused by a single factor, but more than likely is caused by a collection of interactions between the child's internal development and his or her constantly changing environment (Fox, Curry, Pellegrini, Liden). Knowing the crucial nature of interpretation and the complexities of interpretation, the articles in this section focus on the behaviors which should be observed and strongly considered for assessment. Some of these behaviors are cited in the first paragraph.

Theoretically, the intervention strategies which follow assessment and interpretation can be easily managed by teachers and parents (Yawkey). Other strategies become complex, as frequently it is necessary to refer the child to other agencies for further assessment, diagnosis and treatment. Intervention strategies at this level are complicated by diverse referral and diverse financial policies which exist among various agencies and which, on many occasions, prevent the child from ever receiving treatment (Mennis).

Hovering on top of this continuum of "From Recognition to Treatment" are core issues such as the background, experience, and maturity of the professional(s) involved, the indecision that exists around the selection of the appropriate assessment procedures, the correct selection of treatment (VanderVen), the ethical issues that surround labelling, and the legal issues of confidentiality that are passed-down from the federal government (Morrissey). These issues are constantly interplaying in the total assessment and treatment of the "puzzling child."

The editors wish to acknowledge, with deep gratitude, the expertise given by Nancy Curry, Sarah Arnaud, Carole McNamee, William Isler, Carol Cartwright, and Gilbert Foley in many open dialogues which ultimately provided the structure and contents of this issue.

MIF

PUZZLING CHILDREN: A CHALLENGE TO THE CHILD CARE SERVICE SYSTEM

Karen VanderVen, PhD

ABSTRACT. Puzzling children, perhaps much more so than those whose impairments are obvious and for whom there are clearly identified treatments, seem to surface crucial issues in the service delivery system. These encompass such areas as parent-professional relationships; theoretical concepts of etiology and professional discipline; assessment and diagnosis; clinician characteristics, and treatment trends. These issues and their implications for better serving "puzzling" children are described in this paper.

"Such a complicated, puzzling little boy." (Wilson, 1968, p. 38)
"Diagnosis is a very tricky business." (Park, 1976, p. 32)

Who Are the Puzzling Children?

Within the extreme poles of the dimension of normality to exceptionality in children, there lies a gray area of ambiguity within which are contained the puzzling children. These are the children of whom it is difficult for both parents and professionals to determine whether some aspect of their development or behavior is reason for real concern and further action. "How do you recognize the symptoms?

Karen VanderVen is Professor, Child Development and Child Care, University of Pittsburgh, Pittsburgh, PA 15261.

When can you be sure?'' (Lorenz, 1969, p. 20). ''So when did it begin?'' (Park, 1967, p. 21). These are comments made by parents of puzzling children who have written of their experiences raising them. ''He'll grow out of it'' or ''Why did you not seek help sooner?'' are the kinds of statements that professionals may make after studying a puzzling child.

Puzzling children, perhaps much more so than those whose impairments are obvious and for whom there are clearly identified treatments, seem to surface crucial issues in the service delivery system. Like any human enterprise this has, along with its valuable strengths, deficiencies which diminish its effectiveness. These encompass such issues as parent-professional relationships; theoretical concepts of etiology and professional discipline; assessment and diagnosis; clinician characteristics; and treatment trends. Puzzling children, due to the very perplexities and uncertainties that they pose, would seem to be particularly vulnerable to lacks in the service system. Failure to deal effectively with these children can not only lead to a decrease in the probability of their achieving a positive and optimal development, but also to serious tragedy. Because of this, it is essential that these issues be studied and addressed.

Parents and Professionals

One of most core issues is the relationship between parents and professionals, since parents are usually the first to suspect ''that there might be something wrong'' with their child (Featherstone, 1980, p. 13). Following a painful internal debate fueled both by positive and disquieting observations, they may finally consult a professional who may, not always correctly, confirm or allay their fears. Once these contacts have been made, parents have entered an area which exposes them to the vulnerabilities of professionals and the systems in which they work. Unfortunately, many—although certainly not all—professionals have been highly insensitive in their dealings with parents, as has been well documented in their accounts (Featherstone, 1980; Lorenz, 1969; Park, 1967; Wechsler, 1972; Wilson, 1969). Parents report that they are not *listened* to; that their observations are ignored; that there is little concern for the strain they experience in living with a difficult or puzzling child (Brown, 1979).

Probably the greatest lack in parent-professional interaction has been the assignment of blame, either implicitly or explicitly, by professionals, Louise Wilson reports just one of many such comments made to her and her husband as they sought treatment for their puzzling son: 'Certainly you are not *well.* Every child born is...an empty slate. What is written on it... *you* wrote there'' (1968, p. 40). Since, as Featherstone (1980) points out, parents already feel guilt, it seems hardly necessary to reinforce it further, particularly because such guilt can actually then contribute to parental perplexity and even a self-fulfilling prophecy (Thomas and Birch, 1977).

Fortunately, there has been a shift in recent years towards recognizing that, as crucial as parents obviously are as influences on their children's development, there are others too, so that the tendency to ''blame'' parents is gradually diminishing. There has also been a trend, perhaps fueled by the growing number of effective advocacy groups organized around various children's disabilities, to involve, rather than shut parents out of, efforts to assess and treat their children's problems. They are viewed as collaborators rather than adversaries. This promising and constructive orientation needs to continue.

Theoretical Issues

Naturally, there are numerous theoretical issues underlying the approaches taken to working with children. Two that are particularly germane to the challenge of ''puzzling children'' are concepts of causation and the theoretical backgrounds of practitioners. For many years, the field of child development was dominated by a linear model of cause and effect which, as already has been stated, affected attitudes towards parents, in line with Whittaker's (1976) description of ''the family etiology hypothesis.'' Because it also related to choice of assessment procedures and treatments, however, it is highly possible that it contributed towards overly restricted, and hence less effective interventions. For this reason, it is important that the implications of more recent work germane to cause and effect be examined and applied.

Individual differences in constitutional basic temperament (Segal and Yahraes, 1978), exemplified by work such as that of Thomas and Chess (1977), have been shown to be a significant influence, in interaction with the environment, on the courses of children's development. Unusual sensitivities present from birth (Bergman and Escalona, 1949) can play a similar role. Inborn predispositions in children such as these cause them to contribute towards determining the way their families and others in their environment come to treat them, in line with the evidence presented by Bell and Harper (1977) that children indeed influence their caregivers in the same way that caregivers have an influence upon children. The growing field of child ecology establishes that there is a hierarchy of variables affecting children which include but also transcend their immediate environment. All of these factors contribute to the concept of the "interactional" (Magnussen, 1977; Park, 1976, p. 130) approach to consideration of cause and effect in children's development and behavior. This implies that children must be studied from multiple, rather than singular perspectives, and that these be incorporated in the determination of sufficient assessment and treatment methods.

The professional background of the various mental health and developmental practitioners obviously influences the kind of treatments they select. In the case of children it has been shown that professional identity is related to ways of responding to them (Arthur and Birnbaum, 1968). Because there are numerous discrete theoretical persuasions in the disciplines serving children, it is again possible in cases requiring a broad and complex perspective, that a more singular approach reflective of the clinician's particular discipline can contribute to a failure to take relevant variables into account. This issue, obviously, is not an easy one to resolve because there are limitations that are legitimate in the amount of knowledge that can be included in any one discipline, incorporated by any one practitioner, and even considered by a multidisciplinary team of professionals. But the relationship of professional discipline to actual practice needs to be borne in mind.

Diagnostic Issues

The formal identification of problems of a "puzzling child" is usually determined through some kind of diagnostic and assessment process. However, technical deficiencies and inappropriate utilization of the diagnostic period can lead to painful errors. There are dozens of assessment and diagnostic instruments available for studying all kinds of children's problems, and these obviously can provide exceedingly useful information. But it has been shown that such factors as the validity of assessment instruments, the appropriateness of their selection for particular cases, the knowledge and skill of the examiner, and particularly the interpretations and applications of their results, can have deleterious effects, with the needs of particular children not being properly identified or met (Mearig, 1978). Fischer (in Mearig, 1978) points up another important concern, which is that adherence to the formal standardization process can often eliminate the pursuit of crucial clinical information.

These cautions do not suggest that there should be fewer attempts at gathering diagnostic information, even though there seems to be a disquieting and growing trend in this direction (Strupp, 1969). For example, in the area of family therapy, treatment sometimes begins before or without a period of more formal assessment (Bush, 1980). The need for accurate and comprehensive assessment procedures is heightened by the fact that inadequate assessment leads to poor treatment selection which in turn is related to negative outcomes (Strupp, 1969). Such outcomes are a high price to pay if they can be prevented by careful assessment initially.

The clinical decision making process is another important concern in accurate assessment and treatment planning. The complexities of this process have been recognized and attempts have been made to identify variables related to its accuracy (Goldberg, 1968; Oskamp, 1965; Tversky and Kahneman, 1974). Work still needs to be done to determine what information is important, what influences its quality and accuracy, what ways it should be gathered, and in how it should be utilized. Since the effectiveness of decisions has great implications for the kind of interventions that will be selected, it is important that study of the decision making process continue.

Clinician Characteristics

First hand accounts by parents of puzzling children indicate the tremendous range of approaches and responses that were reflected by a spectrum of professionals encountered in long searches for help (Featherstone, 1980; Lorenz, 1969; Park, 1967; Wechsler, 1972). The fact that clinicians, like children, proceed through their own stages of professional development from immaturity to maturity (Stoltenberg, 1980; Burton, 1972) has tremendous implications for working for and with children who have complex, subtle difficulties. Younger, more inexperienced professionals who nonetheless are practicing are less likely to have the breadth of knowledge and the cognitive complexity to grasp and work with the multiple variables that may be significant.

For example, Gordon (1980) describes how his perspectives towards his therapeutic approaches changed "full circle" as he practiced over the years and incorporated new knowledge and ongoing experience into his work. In these days of reduced resources, it is hard to insist that all clinicians providing assessment and treatment be at their highest level of professional maturity. On the other hand, it does need to be recognized that the effectiveness of services can be seriously compromised if they are delivered by those with a too narrow perspective or unrefined treatment skills.

Unpleasant as it is, it must also be taken into consideration that some professionals may let their own personal dynamics affect the quality of the service they deliver; effects from "negative countertransference" are another variable associated, not surprisingly, with poor outcomes in treatment (Strupp, 1969). While some training programs for clinicians encourage awareness of the possibility of the practitioners' personal reactions having a deleterious effect on their clients, not all do. The parents' accounts poignantly underscore the devastating effects of what would seem to be unjustifiably harsh responses. This certainly implies that self-awareness is a crucial aspect in the preparation and continuing education of any clinician.

Treatment Trends

Child treatment, like any other discipline or activity, is affected by shifting trends. These, of course, are necessary in order to advance the field and scope of practice. It is important, on the other hand, that these not be overemphasized to the total exclusion of other relevant perspectives and approaches. Two well-known focuses of current practice are family therapy and early intervention, to name a few which are particularly relevant to puzzling children.

Few would dispute that treatment effectiveness has been greatly extended by the shift towards systems theory and family vs. individual treatment (Roman and Blackburn, 1979). However, it has been pointed out that this can, in some cases, be misapplied and overapplied. Important variables, such as those contributed by the child himself, can be ignored, thereby compromising the breadth of the treatment (McDermott and Char, 1974).

Early intervention is another practice which has been strongly emphasized, with the contention that early identification of, and action on, developing problems can prevent them from becoming more serious or entrenched later. It has been pointed out that early identification usually involves labeling a child, and that while labels may be necessary in order to secure proper treatment, they may also stigmatize and lead into securing inappropriate interventions (Hobbs, 1975). A skeptical perspective on early intervention and labeling is found in the provocative book *The Myth of the Hyperactive Child* (Schrag and Divoky, 1975). Focusing on children who have been termed "hyperactive," "learning disabled," "minimally brain damaged" etc., the authors suggest that certain interventions, such as drug therapy, have been inappropriately used on these children, on the premise that they may not really be in need of special treatment. Rather, the interventions are applied because others happen to find their behavior annoying. Because "puzzling" children may be among those who are discussed in this book, the issue it poses is relevant. However, it would seem that the core concern is not whether there should be early identification of children with such disorders, because there is extensive evidence that they do exist and that they can lead to serious difficulties in later life if left unrecognized. Rather, it would seem that it would be with ensuring that the assessment is accurate, so that differentiation can be made, with each individual, between behavior which is simply annoying and that which is leading the child into a course of negative development.

Eileen Simpson, a dyslexic, describes her painful childhood which perplexed both herself and others. In *Reversals* (1979) she states that 'throughout my childhood and youth the nature of my disorder remained mysterious to me and those in my milieu. When I was twenty-two it was diagnosed—not by a psychologist but by a poet: I was dyslexic" (p. vii).

Solving the challenges posed by "puzzling" children such as Mrs. Simpson was and will not be easy. Some of the possible relevant issues have been identified which hopefully will encourage this task.

REFERENCES

Arthur, B., & Birnbaum, J. Professional identity as a determinant of the response to emotionally disturbed children. *Psychiatry,* 1968, *31*, 138-149

Aponte, H. Family therapy and the community. In M. Gibbs, J. Lachenmeyer, & J. Sigal (Eds.), *Community psychology*. New York: Gardner Press, Inc., 1980.

Bell, R., & Harper, L. *Child effects on adults*. Hillsdale, New Jersey: Lawrence Erlbaum Associates, 1977.

Bergman, P., & Escalona, S. Unusual sensitivities in very young children. *Psychoanalytic study of the child*, 1949, *3*, 333-352.

Bolman, W. Obstacles to prevention. *The basic handbook of child psychiatry* (Vol. IV). New York: Basic Books, 1979, 8-12.
Broskowski, A., & Baker, F. Professional, organizational and social barriers to primary prevention. *Amer. J. Orthopsychiatry*, 1974, *44*, 707-719.
Brown, S. Assuring due process in special educational placement and the roles of child and youth service professionals. *Child and youth services*, 1979, *4*, 1-11.
Burton, A., & Associates. *Twelve therapists*. San Francisco: Jossey-Bass, 1972.
Bush, R. *A parents' guide to child therapy*. New York: Delacorte Press, 1980.
Featherstone, H. *A difference in the family*. New York: Basic Books, 1980.
Gauron, E.D. Diagnostic decision making in psychiatry. *Archives Gen. Psychiatry*, 1966, *14*, 225-232.
Goldberg, L. Simple models or simple processes: Some research on clinical judgments. *American Psychologist*, 1968, *23*, 483-496.
Gordon, E. The making of a target child. *The Family*, 1980, *8*, 30-35.
Hobbs, N. *The futures of children*. San Francisco: Jossey-Bass, 1975.
Lorenz, S. *Our son Ken*. New York: Dell Publishing Co., 1969.
Magnussen, D., & Endler, N. Interactional psychology: Present status and future prospects. In D. Magnussen & N. Endler (Eds.), *Personality at the crossroads: Current issues in interactional psychology*. New Jersey: Lawrence Erlbaum, 1977.
McDermott, J., & Char, W. The undeclared war between child and family therapy. *Journal of the American Academy of Child Psychiatry*, 1974, *13*, 422-436.
Mearig, J., & Associates. *Working for children: Ethical issues beyond professional guidelines*. San Francisco: Jossey-Bass, 1978.
Oskamp, S. Overconfidence in case-study judgments. *Journal of Consulting Psychology*, 1965, *29*, 261-265.
Park, C. *The siege*. New York: Harcourt, Brace & World, 1967.
Park, C., & Shapiro, L. *You are not alone*. Boston: Little Brown, 1976.
Roman, M., & Blackburn, S. *Family secrets*. New York: Times Books, 1979.
Schrag, P., & Divoky, D. *The myth of the hyperactive child*. New York: Pantheon, 1975.
Segal, H., & Yahraes, H. *A child's journey: Forces that shape the lives of our young*. New York: McGraw-Hill, 1978.
Simpson, E. *Reversals*. Boston: Houghton Mifflin, 1979.
Sines, L. The relative contribution of four kinds of data to the accuracy of personality assessment. *Journal of Consulting Psychology*, 1959, *23*, 483-492.
Skolnick, A. The myth of the vulnerable child. *Psychology Today*, February, 1978, 56-65.
Stoltenberg, C. Approaching supervision from a developmental perspective: The counselor complexity model. *Journal of Counseling Psychology*, 1981, *28*, 59-65.
Strupp, H., Hadley, S., & Gomes-Schwartz, B. *Psychotherapy for better or worse: The problem of negative effects*. New York: Jason Aronson, 1977.
Strupp, H., Fox, R., & Lessler, K. *Patients view their psychotherapy*. Baltimore: The Johns Hopkins Press, 1969.
Thomas, A., & Chess, S. *Temperament and development*. New York: Brunner/Mazel, 1977.
Tversky, A., & Kahneman, D. Judgment under uncertainty: Heuristics and biases. *Science*, 1974, *185*, 1124-1131.
Wechsler, J. *In a darkness*. New York: W.W. Norton, 1972.
Whittaker, J. Causes of childhood disorders: New findings. *Social Work*, 1976, *21*, 91-96.
Wilson, S. Journey of a lost boy. *Look Magazine*, February 6 and 20, 1968.

THE PRINCIPLES OF OBSERVATION

Gilbert M. Foley, EdD

ABSTRACT. Observational data are essential in unraveling the complexity of the puzzling child. This paper presents broad orienting principles to serve as a framework for both the observer and the process of observation.

Meticulous observation is the foundation of all developmental assessment in children and a common denominator in almost all scientific and clinical work. The universality of observation makes it a skill of central importance to scientists and clinicians alike. For those desiring greater insight into the developmental processes of children, observational skills are a sine qua non.

The following are broad principles to serve as a framework for both the observer and the process of observation.

I. The good observer is able to use a variety of settings and varying degrees of structure to collect a representative sample of behavior.

Almost everything the child does is telling whether it be in the home, classroom or clinic. The child projects his own style, tempo and

Gilbert M. Foley is Project Director, Family Centered Resource Project, Berks County Intermediate Unit, and Clinical Instructor of Pediatrics, Medical College of Pennsylvania, 1251 Eckert Avenue, Reading, PA 19602.

This work was developed in part under a grant from the U.S. Department of Education No. G007802653 (Office of Special Education). The content does not necessarily reflect the position or policy of that Agency, and no official endorsement of these materials should be inferred.

character onto the most mundane activities, "the symbolics of everyday life," thus providing a screen for reading the emerging personality. Motor skills can be observed in the planning required to get a drink as well as in the activities of gym. Cognitive skills such as memory, discrimination and synthesis can be gleaned from watching and listening to a child relate to his teacher during storytime as well as from the results of a paper and pencil test.

A sample of behavior can be collected in a completely naturalistic way by observing the child proceed through his daily routine or structuring a specific set of environmental variables or stimuli. Thus the good observer should be able to function comfortably on the structural continuum knowing when to focus or expand stimuli and situations in order to better understand the child. Of course, the good observer must know what to look for, be a sensitive cue reader and possess a cognitive map to sort and organize observed data.

II . The good observer maintains a state of dynamic balance between empathy and distance.

Empathy involves the ability to feel oneself into another's phenomenology or experience and provides the observer with an intimate glimpse and understanding of the world of the observed. For this state to occur, there must be an openness on the part of the professional resulting in a partial and temporary identification with the client (Korchin, 1976).

The common themes of human experience such as love, loss, and grief frequently act as catalytic agents of the empathic state. Yet, empathy must be balanced with distance, for overidentification and fusion with the client interfere with the professional's powers of judgment (Schafer, 1959). Too much distance likewise inhibits the closeness necessary for the sharing of experience and interpersonal understanding.

III. The good observer records the data systematically and objectively and communicates them articulately.

The observational protocol must consist of behaviors and not inferences or interpretations of behavior. The recording should be simple and clear. Attention should be paid to both the social context and temporal sequences of the observed data. Thus, Taguiri (1969, p. 420) notes: " 'The boy *began* to *sob*, then he hit his playmate in the face' gives the act of beginning to sob a different meaning from 'The boy hit his playmate in the face, then he *began to sob*.' "

The affective state and needs of both the observer and the observed greatly influence the kind of inferences that might be made from the raw data and should be identified. The hungry person is alerted to food. Individuals in a state of fright are more likely to perceive others as more fearful or aggressive (Feshbach & Singer, 1957).

Vigilance must also be exercised by the observer to avoid over-simplication and reduction of the amount of information into unitary or stereotyped descriptions.

IV. The good observer has theoretical frames of reference to serve as a basis for interpretation and considers competing hypotheses.

When a representative sample of behavior has been collected and carefully recorded, the process of synthesis and analysis is commenced.

In this task, it is imperative that interpretations not be based on any single indicator. Rather, recurrent patterns and central themes, red-threads that weave themselves through the protocol, should be identified and serve as the basis for interpretive work (Saul, 1972).

For example, the preschool child observed propping to maintain stability, holding on to change position, leaning into the desk for support and resisting to cross midline manually during the course of a typical day, presents a pattern of indicators suggestive of a gross motor planning problem. While the sample may not be sufficient for making a differential diagnosis, it is a valid basis for referral for more extensive evaluation. It is also a basis for beginning functional intervention and suggests that the child needs greater central control through positioning to achieve the stability necessary to meet the related challenges of preschool.

When observing young children or analyzing observational protocols, it is also important to be sensitive to behaviors that demonstrate the interaction between developmental domains. Because development is a simultaneous and interactive process and the young child is still not significantly domain differentiated, a dysfunction in one domain is likely to have secondary negative impact on related domains. As a result, identifying these juncture points may be more useful than determining levels of function within domains.

Naturalistic observation is most useful in this respect for it permits us to see the child in his complexity employing the full range of his adaptive capacity.

While interviewing the mother of an infant designated as "at-risk," she expressed grave concern that her child had no "emotions." After a physical therapist and I observed and played with the child, we realized he was severely hypotonic and did not have the muscular capability of forming highly differentiated facial expressions. This child's motor problem inhibited normal baby-mother reciprocity precipitating a mild disturbance in attachment and the mother's perception of her infant as emotionless. Establishing this motor-emotional relationship not only provided great relief to the mother, who harbored fears that her child did not know or like her, but provided a viable point for intervention.

V. The good observer has theoretical frames of reference to serve as a basis for interpretation and considers competing hypotheses.

Human development is the counterpoint between lawfulness and uniqueness. The good observer must be thoroughly grounded in the principles, milestones and temporal parameters of normal human development. This nomothetic (Allport, 1937) orientation is the referent, the zero point against which to make quantitative judgments regarding the normalcy of a child's observed behavior.

Likewise, the good observer needs to have a knowledge of individual differences and human uniqueness. This is developed by extensive clinical experience with individual students or clients. The idiographic orientation (Allport, 1937) is the referent for assessing quality of function and individual style.

Frequently it is assessment of quality that makes the difference between identifying or missing the subtly involved child. The mildly learning disabled child may complete all the age appropriate tasks but with considerable effort, efficiency reducing compensations and complications in related domains. The sensitive observer with a good "clinical eye" will identify the child, secure appropriate services and prevent the cumulative dysfunctions that would likely develop.

A behavior such as hyperactivity can be symptomatic of a variety of etiological factors. When the observer interprets such behaviors he should have thorough knowledge of various clinical and theoretical explanations and test competing hypothesis against the observed data before assuming any one differential diagnosis. At all costs the Procrustian Propensity must be avoided, i.e., the urge to make the data fit any given theory.

VI. The good observer knows himself.

All observational data are potentially influenced by the characterological style of the observer. Our individual defense structures may determine that we see a conflict-free world or a jungle, a tragic scenario or a romantic epic. Knowledge of oneself reduces the risks of observer error, by acting as a cognitive censor against such pitfalls as projection, characterological response sets, biased attitudes, oversimplification and selective perception.

Observing with psychological self-mindedness, an "intrapsychic eye," contributes to the potential richness of both the data collection and interpretive processes. Self-insight allows one to bring the distilled complexity of his own personality, associative repertoire, and uniqueness into the observational area. This enhances the sensitivity of the observer to perceive and respect the differentiated complexity of others.

Good judges of personality tend to possess a variety of intellectual traits and personality qualities which enhance their accuracy of person perception. Korchin's review of the literature (1976) indicates that intelligence, breadth of experience, cognitive complexity, psychological mindedness and personal insight are among the most salient traits. "In general, the more intellectually limited the observer is or the more restricted in depth and breadth of personality, the more likely is he to lack skill in judging another person" (Korchin, 1976, p. 153).

BIBLIOGRAPHY

Allport, G.W. *Personality: A psychological interpretation*. New York: Holt, 1937.
Feshbach, S., & Singer, R.D. The effects of fear arousal and suppression of fear upon social perception. *Journal of Abnormal and Social Psychology*, 1957, *55*, 283-288.
Korchin, S.J. *Modern clinical psychology*. New York: Basic Books, 1976.
Saul, L. *Psycho-dynamically based psychotherapy*. New York: Science House, 1972.
Schafer, R. Generative empathy in the treatment situation. *Psychoanalytic Quarterly*, 1959, *28*, 342-373.
Taguiri, R. Person perception. In G. Lindzey and E. Aronson (Eds.), *The handbook of social psychology*, Vol. III (2nd ed.) Reading, Mass.: Addison-Wesley, 1969.

OBSERVATION TECHNIQUES

Carol A. Cartwright, PhD
Cecelia B. Ward

ABSTRACT. This is a "how-to-do-it" treatment of observation methods. Major steps in the observation process are described and important general guidelines for accurate observation and record keeping are provided. Procedures for controlling error and improving the efficiency of observation processes are included. Record keeping by using anecdotal records, running records, checklists, participation charts, charting and tallying behaviors, and rating scales is described. For each type of record, advantages and disadvantages, procedures for designing forms, suggested uses, and tips on interpreting data are included. A brief summary section focuses on the role of observation in identification and diagnosis.

Observation was the primary tool for documenting and understanding children's behavior during the child study movement that was popular in the U.S. in the 1920s and 1930s. Gradually, other research techniques and data collection procedures, especially tests, were favored, and it was not until the 1960s and 1970s that we experienced a revival of interest in the value of naturalistic observation. As scientists and teachers understood more thoroughly the complex nature of human behavior and the influence of the physical and social context on behavior, they realized the unique contributions of observation.

Carol A. Cartwright is Professor of Education, The Pennsylvania State University, and Cecelia B. Ward is a PhD candidate at The Pennsylvania State University, University Park, PA 16802.

The purpose of this article is to describe major steps in the observation process and to set forth general considerations in observation and record keeping. Various types of records, along with their advantages and disadvantages, and tips on using procedures and interpreting information are included. In other words, this is the "nuts and bolts" article in this volume.

The Observation Process

Observation is a process of systematically looking at and recording behavior for the purpose of making instructional decisions (Cartwright and Cartwright, 1974). Accurate observational data are essential for the interpretation, identification, diagnosis and treatment of specific behaviors. In fact, much of the information about children that is of interest to us is not obtainable in any other way except through observation.

Irwin and Bushnell (1980) view observation as an important part of the teaching process for the following reasons:

1. It is a means of generating ideas about children.
2. It is a means of answering specific questions about a particular child or the class as a whole.
3. Observation provides a more realistic view of behavior than do other methods of information gathering.
4. It may help us to better understand children's behavior.
5. It functions as a means of evaluation either of a group of children or an individual child.

According to Cartwright and Cartwright (1974) observation serves a variety of functions. It can supplement other information, which is crucial when comprehensive information is needed. Observation is useful for making decisions about appropriate objectives, methods, and materials for instruction. Finally, important characteristics of individual children can be identified through observation, including the early detection of problems.

Even though observation is useful for a variety of purposes, there are several basic, or common, steps involved in all types of observation: (1) determine the purpose; (2) choose the type of record and design the form; (3) collect data; (4) summarize and interpret data. Each step will be explained in more detail. Space does not permit inclusion of examples of record forms, but each of the references given is an excellent source of many examples and interested readers are encouraged to consult them.

Purpose of the Observation—Key to Additional Decisions

Because the purpose of the observation has implications for all aspects of the observation process, the observer must be quite clear on why the observation is taking place. If the purpose is well defined, it will determine the answers to the following questions:

1. Who will make the observation?
2. Who or what will be observed?
3. Where will the observation take place? (there should be a variety of situations included).
4. When will the observation occur? (there should be diversified time periods).
5. How will the observation be recorded? (Cartwright and Cartwright, 1974).

General Considerations in Observation and Record Keeping

The choice of a recording procedure must be based on the purpose for the observation. Some types of records are easier to use, while others may result in more objective and reliable information. However, if the type of record chosen does not match the purpose of the observation, the choice is inappropriate and the information may be of questionable value.

A certain amount of time and effort is required to develop and use observational records. In fact, there is often a trade-off between the amount of time spent in development and the amount of time needed to use and interpret a type of record. What must be kept in mind throughout the development of observational records is that our ultimate goal is a record that allows us to gather information objectively.

An essential element of objectivity is an operational definition of the behavior of interest. The behavior being observed and documented should be described so specifically that any time any child displays the behavior it can easily be determined whether or not the behavior has occurred. Examples of different instances of the behavior are an extremely useful way of adding precision to a definition. Other means of increasing objectivity include experimenting with the record form, to revise and improve it, practicing using the form, and having other observers independently record their observations to check on observer agreement (Cartwright and Cartwright, 1974).

Even though considerable thought and effort may go into the choice and preparation of a recording procedure, errors may still occur. It is possible to limit the amount of error in the observation process through training and practice with the methods. Also, the accuracy of observation can be checked by having several people observe the children or events independently and then they can check on their agreement with each other. The better the agreement, the more objective is the observation. Taking care to be selective in the choice of behaviors to be observed and in the amount of information collected will also help to control errors, especially for beginners. Other ways to control errors are to make the record while the observation is being conducted, if possible, and to gather observations at a variety of times and situations. For certain problems it may be necessary to concentrate observations on certain children or certain behaviors. In general, teachers will want to take care to get samples of different behaviors from all children though.

Although there are certain inherent tendencies and biases in observers which influence and introduce error into the observation process, these sources of bias can be controlled. A conscious attempt by the observer to reduce and eliminate bias is one helpful procedure. For example, a teacher who thinks a particular child is "cute" will need to guard carefully to be sure that observations are not positive because of the idea of cuteness but accurately reflect what behaviors are really being displayed. A word of caution about observational information must be inserted. Although errors can be controlled, they can never be eliminated. Therefore, our interpretation of observational information should be tentative and all conclusions need to be checked continually.

Irwin and Bushnell's (1980) observation guidelines reinforce and add to the preceding information.

1. Describe in writing the purpose and procedure of your observation.
2. It is usually desirable to select an unobtrusive vantage point for observing.
3. Information gathered on individual children should be treated confidentially.

4. Be as objective as possible; avoid letting your own feelings about the subject of your observation color or slant your observations.
5. Include the following information on every record you use: identity of observer; name of child or description of event; date and time of observation; the setting or location.
6. Draw only conclusions which can be justified by the observational information.

Observation is a time-consuming process but there are ways to use observation time more efficiently. One way of improving the efficiency of collecting observational data is by making observation a habit, a routine part of what you do as a teacher. In general, the more you use observational methods, the more efficient you become, both in their use and in your use of time.

A variety of strategies and aids are available that improve accuracy as well as efficiency of observation. Index cards, small notebooks, clipboards, and copies of various recording forms can be kept in convenient places throughout the classroom so that an observation can be recorded as it is observed. Portable tape recorders are an efficient way of unobtrusively capturing children's conversations. For those situations involving tallying frequencies of behavior or time—sampling procedures, a variety of inexpensive counters and timers—golfer's wrist watch, supermarket counter, kitchen timer—are available. Simple shorthand or coding systems can be devised to record information rapidly. Photographs, movie films, videotapes can also be used if the equipment is available (Cartwright, Cartwright, and Ward, 1981).

Types of Records

Anecdotal Records and Running Records

Anecdotal records are brief accounts of some event that happened—a "word picture" of a behavior or incident. To be useful, anecdotal records must be factual; interpretations are not a part of the record form. Anecdotal records are appropriately used for spontaneous, unexpected behaviors, incidents, or events and therefore need to be open-ended. They should not be used for behaviors that can be anticipated in advance. However, they are invaluable for documenting unanticipated behaviors that are not likely to be included in other kinds of records.

The most important consideration in the preparation of anecdotal records is assuring that the information recorded is factual. The observer should record exactly what happened in an objective way and should write down the information at the time the observation is occurring. Each anecdotal record should be limited to a description of one specific incident and any interpretation should be kept separate from the incident itself.

The observer's biases can easily be reflected in anecdotal records. This can occur in the choice of behaviors to be recorded as well as the language used to describe the behavior. One way of eliminating some of the subjectivity of anecdotal records is to use one word or phrase consistently to describe a behavior. Providing supporting information, such as samples of work, may also cut down on observer bias.

It is important to prepare a general format for the recording of anecdotal information. Important information is less likely to be forgotten and the information is more likely to be recorded systematically. Certain items must be included on an anecdotal record: the name of the child, the name of the observer, the time and setting at which the incident occurred, and a space for the description of the incident itself (Cartwright and Cartwright, 1974).

Even though the behaviors recorded in anecdotal records are unexpected, decisions on what to record should be made in terms of some specific purpose. You should also have some plan for collecting anecdotal data in order to handle the large volume of information and to insure that all children are included. For example, you may decide to prepare at least one anecdotal record for some child during free play each day. Or you may systematically go through your class list, preparing an anecdotal record for a set number of children each day.

Interpretation of anecdotal records should wait until several anecdotes about the same child are available so patterns may emerge. This interpretation needs to be kept separate from the recording of the incident. Therefore, we recommend that anecdotes be summarized and interpretations made on separate forms. In this way, you will be better able to determine if the behaviors recorded represent typical behaviors for that child and if patterns can be discerned. Recommendations for further action, a consultation or referral for example, may be included on the summary sheet.

Running records are quite similar to anecdotal records but are generally more complete. They try to capture the most important elements of a behavior or event in as much detail as possible. The observer usually keeps a running record over an extended period of time, rather than simply recording an incident and then not recording for minutes, hours, or days. The intent is to record the situation in a manner that lets someone else read the description later and visualize the event as it occurred (Irwin and Bushnell, 1980). The same principles and cautions that guide the development and interpretation of anecdotal records apply to running records.

Checklists and Participation Charts

A checklist consists of a list of expected behaviors, together with a space for recording whether the items are present or not. Checklists should be used when the behaviors to be observed are known in advance and there is no need for information about the quality characteristics or the frequency of the behavior. This lack of information about quality and frequency is the major disadvantage of checklists.

An advantage of using a checklist is that a great deal of information can be recorded quickly. Another advantage is that, since the behaviors of interest are specified in advance, you will probably not overlook some essential behavior. Checklists require a simple yes-no checkmark response on the part of the observer, and therefore allow little room for observer bias.

In general, the starting point for developing a checklist will be the behavioral objectives of the program. The objectives, if clearly defined, can be simply translated into items on the checklist. Developmental milestones are another appropriate starting point for checklists, particularly when the identification of developmental problems is the purpose of the observation. Variations or deviations from the anticipated behavior can be recorded, along with the expected behavior. The listing of behaviors should be in a logical order to increase the efficiency of the observation. In areas where learning outcomes may be slow or occur over a long period of time, the date rather than a checkmark can be inserted next to the statement of the behavior exhibited. Items should describe a single behavior unless you are certain all parts of the item will be learned at the same time.

In summary, the guidelines for developing a checklist are:

1. The checklist must be prepared before the observation.
2. List the target behaviors separately on the checklist.
3. The checklist should be logically organized.
4. The organization of the checklist should meet all the stated purposes of the observation (Irwin and Bushnell, 1980).

Participation charts are similar to checklists in that they are used to record the presence or absence of behaviors. However, they are used to record the behaviors of many learners simultaneously, when participation in some activity is the behavior of interest. Most participation charts consist of a list of the names of the children and a space to tally each child's participation. The form should also include spaces for the type of activity, the date, and the name of the observer. The format could also be set up to correspond to the seating arrangement in use during the activity.

Behavior Tallying and Charting

One of the simplest ways to record behaviors as they are occurring is to tally each instance of the behavior. Frequency counts are appropriate for behaviors that are discrete units and that occur fairly infrequently during a day. The behavior must be clearly defined in observable terms. Number of math problems completed is an example of a behavior for which a frequency count would be appropriate.

For other behaviors, the relevant information is the amount of time spent performing the behavior or its duration. Crying or temper tantrums are examples of behaviors for which duration might be recorded. As with frequency counts, the behavior must be operationally defined in order for its duration to be recorded accurately. Rate combines both frequency and duration information. The number of times something happens is counted and that number is divided by the amount of time the teacher kept track of it; e.g., number of math problems completed in a 15-minute period of time. This procedure is useful when dealing with frequently occurring behaviors, for which it would be difficult to record all instances of the behavior.

Information about frequency or duration of behavior is easier to interpret if it is transferred to a graph or chart. Graphs should be clearly labeled to indicate the type of behavior recorded, the time period, the observer, and any other information needed to interpret the observations. The number of observation periods (such as days) are recorded on the horizontal axis and the behavior being counted or timed is recorded on the vertical axis. Line graphs are recommended over bar charts because of the ease of preparation and their suitability for showing several behaviors on the same graph.

Rating Scales

Rating scales are similar to checklists in that the expected behaviors are known in advance. They differ in that the observer is asked to rate the quality or frequency of the behavior. Rating scales can be used where it is possible to determine the extent to which a particular quality is present. Usually the behavior to be observed has several different aspects and each aspect is rated on a separate scale. The observer must make a judgment about the frequency or quality characteristics of the behavior.

These judgements can be a source of error. For example, there is a tendency to give higher rating than ought to be given because of a generally favorable attitude toward the child—called the halo effect. Other common rater errors include: (1) error of leniency—rating someone higher than he or she deserves to be rated; (2) error of central tendency—rating everyone toward the middle; (3) error of logic—giving a similar rating to items that seem to be related; (4) proximity error—rating items that are next to each other similarly. Simply being aware of potential errors may help to reduce or eliminate them (Cartwright and Cartwright, 1974; Irwin and Bushnell, 1980).

Despite the potential for error, rating scales do have several advantages. The most obvious is that rating scales are relatively easy to develop and to use, requiring little training. Rating scales provide a basis for comparing children on similar behaviors and direct the observation toward specific dimensions of the behavior. There is also the possibility of pooling ratings from several observers to get an average rating on a child's performance (Cartwright and Cartwright, 1974; Irwin and Bushnell, 1980).

Rating scales can take many forms. However, all share two major components: the list of dimensions of the behaviors which will be rated and the scale(s) which will be used to rate each behavior. The first step in developing a rating scale is to list the important dimensions of the behavior. The dimensions must be directly observable and only one component of the behavior is involved for each rating. The type of scale to be used depends upon the purpose of the observation. The different types of rating scales will be described briefly.

1. Constant alternative scales: The same set of alternatives, descriptive or numerical, are used to rate every dimension of the behavior or each item.
2. Changing alternative scales: Different sets of alternatives are used to rate the different behavior dimensions.
3. Numerical rating scales: The observer marks a number to indicate the degree to which a behavior is present or the quality of the performance. Each of the numbers may be given a verbal description or only the end points of the scale may be described. Numerical rating scales can be constant alternative or changing alternatives.
4. Simple graphic rating scales: A line is drawn and points along the line are identified. The rater may mark anywhere along the line, even between the defined points. Sometimes only the end points will be described. Simple graphic scales can be constant alternative or changing alternatives.
5. Descriptive graphic rating scales: The degree of quality or frequency are specifically described in behavioral terms and the descriptions are placed along a line. These rating scales are usually of the changing alternative type. Descriptive graphic scales generally yield more objective results than other types of rating scales because the specific descriptions tend to be clearer and unidimensional.

Role of Observation in Identification and Diagnosis

Observation plays an important role in the identification and diagnosis of developmental problems of young children. The teacher of young children who is a skilled observer can identify potential problems at an early stage where they can be remediated or controlled. Knowledge of normal developmental milestones provides a standard by which to judge whether an observed behavior or pattern of behaviors is normal or unusual. Developmental milestones are also useful as a source of items for checklists and rating scales. Your knowledge of child development, combined with the observation techniques covered in this article, are powerful tools to evaluate all the children in your classroom.

Teachers are not the only ones who can identify possible developmental problems through observation. Parents are an important source of information about their child and they can often gather observational information at home. By providing them with appropriate recording forms and tips on observation, you can help them in their role of observer. Other sources of observational information are the specialists who may be called into the classroom to aid in the identification and diagnosis of developmental problems. Even the child may be enlisted to help in keeping records of his or her behavior. Young children are capable of maintaining simple behavioral records on their daily activities. By gathering information from a variety of observers, the teacher is better prepared to interpret puzzling behaviors and make recommendations based on factual, comprehensive information rather than hunches or impressions.

REFERENCES

Cartwright, C. A. and Cartwright, G.P. *Developing observation skills*. New York: McGraw-Hill, 1974.

Cartwright, G. P., Cartwright, C. A. and Ward, M. E. *Educating special learners*. Belmont, CA: Wadsworth Publishing Co., 1981.

Irwin, D. M. and Bushnell, M. M. *Observational strategies for child study*. New York: Holt, Rinehart and Winston, 1980.

TEMPERAMENT AND ITS INFLUENCE ON BEHAVIOR

Marian M. Fox, PhD

ABSTRACT. Temperament was defined in terms of the nine behavioral style dimensions and three diagnostic clusters identified by the NYLS researchers. Various assessment instruments were discussed in terms of theoretical framework, format, and psychometric properties. Only one instrument is available for use by teachers. The effects of behavioral style on teachers' perceptions of students were summarized. Teachers' perceptions of children's adaptability levels appear to have far-reaching implications for professional educators.

The recent history of the study of temperament began with the New York Longitudinal Study (NYLS), a comprehensive, ongoing investigation initiated in the late 1950s (Thomas, Chess, Birch, Hertzig, and Korn, 1963). Since that time, the concept of temperament has provided researchers and clinicians with a useful framework for understanding the puzzling child. A body of literature has developed over the last twenty years which incorporates varied aspects of temperament research. Of particular interest are those aspects which relate to the definition and measurement of temperament, and those aspects which deal with the practical significance of temperament research to educators and clinicians.

Temperament, or a synonomous term, behavioral style refers to the

Marian M. Fox is affiliated with Teacher Education at Widener University, Chester, PA 19013.

how of behavior. A description of a child's temperament portrays his/her customary style of interacting with various elements of the environment. For instance, two children may solve an arithmetic problem. Their motive for solving the problem may be similar and their ability to solve the problem may be nearly equal. However, one child may approach the problem in a behavioral style quite different from the other. One child, for example, might appear highly distractible and less persistent. Her attention might be diverted by a minimal amount of extraneous stimuli. These stylistic dimensions of distractibility, attention span-persistence, and threshold of responsiveness constitute part of the temperament profile of the child (Thomas and Chess, 1977).

Through inductive content analyses of parental interviews, the NYLS investigators identified nine temperament variables: activity level, rhythmicity, distractibility, approach-withdrawal, adaptability, persistence, mood, intensity of reaction, and sensory threshold (Thomas et al., 1963). From the interview protocols, each infant was given a score on a 3-point scale on each of the nine variables.

Activity level was defined as the characteristic motor behavior present in the child's functioning. Rhythmicity was defined as the characteristic regularity of the child particularly in terms of biological functioning such as sleeping and eating. Approach-withdrawal dealt with the child's initial response to new situations, while adaptability was defined as the ease with which a routine situation could be altered. Threshold of responsiveness was defined as the intensity level of stimulation necessary to evoke a response from the child. Intensity of reaction referred to the general energy level of a response. Quality of mood referred to the general positive or negative affect of the child. Distractibility was defined as the ease with which a child could be diverted by extraneous environmental stimuli. Attention span-persistence referred to the length of time a child pursued an activity and would continue the activity in the face of obstacles.

In a later investigation Thomas, Chess, and Birch (1977) identified three clusters of temperament characteristics into which approximately 65% of the subjects were classified. These classifications were designated "Difficult," "Easy," and "Slow-to-Warm-Up."

The largest single group was designated as "Easy." These children were characterized as being regular in biological functioning, positive in approach responses, adaptable to change, generally positive in mood, with mild to moderately intense reactions to stimuli. The "Difficult'' child showed irregularity in biological functioning, withdrawal responses of high intensity, nonadaptability, and negative mood. The 'Slow-to-Warm-Up'' child was characterized by slow adaptability, quiet withdrawal and negative responses of mild intensity.

The nine behavioral style variables and the "Difficult," "Easy," and "Slow-to-Warm-Up" constellations identified by the NYLS group have provided the theoretical foundation for many of the assessment instruments which are currently available.

Carey (1970) in an attempt to overcome the lengthy interviewing process of the NYLS, designed a 76-item parent rating scale for use as a screening device for "Difficult" infants in pediatric clinical practice. In an effort to improve its psychometric properties and to increase its effectiveness as a research instrument, the rating scale entitled the Infant Temperament Questionnaire (ITQ) was later revised (Carey and McDevitt, 1978). The revised version of the ITQ contains 95 items, each of which are rated by parents on a 6-point scale. All of the items tap the nine temperament dimensions identified by the NYLS.

The development of the ITQ inspired the subsequent development of similar parent questionnaires. The Toddler Temperament Scale (TTS) is now available to assess the temperament characteristics of children from 1 to 3 years of age (Note 1). The Behavioral Style Questionnaire (BSQ) was developed to assess the temperament characteristics of children from 3 to 7 years of age (McDevitt and Carey, 1978). Most recently, an assessment instrument for children 8 to 12 years of age has been completed (Note 2).

The ITQ, the TTS, and the BSQ share similar characteristics. Items on all three instruments were written to correspond to the nine temperament variables of the NYLS. Each is designed to be completed by parents. Items are written so that the behavioral descriptions are couched within a specific, observable context. The statements are worded to pertain to specific activities and are behaviorally defined. For example, "The child had trouble leaving the mother the first three days when he/she entered school" (BSQ). All of the items are arranged on a Likert-type scale with choices ranging from "almost never" to "almost always." Respectable psychometric properties have been reported for all three instruments (Carey, 1981).

Thomas and Chess (1977) have adapted their own interview process into a parent questionnaire format appropriate for the assessment of children 3 to 7 years of age. The statements are behaviorally defined and can be answered on a 7-point scale from "hardly ever" to "almost always." For instance, "When upset or annoyed with a task my child may throw it down, cry, yell or slam the door, etc." (Thomas and Chess, 1977). In addition to the Parent Questionnaire, Thomas and Chess have developed a Teacher Temperament Questionnaire appropriate for the assessment of children 3 to 7 years of age within the classroom setting. The characteristics of this instrument are similar to those of the Parent Questionnaire. No reliability or validity data are currently available for these instruments.

Other assessment instruments to measure temperament characteristics have been developed independently of the NYLS group (Buss and Plomin, 1975; Rowe and Plomin, 1977). However, the primary objective of this research has been to explore the question of heritability.

Until recently, relatively little attention has been paid to the relationship of behavioral style to school adjustment and academic achievement. Bell (1968) in a review of maternal-child behavior studies argued that the child's characteristics were important determinants of the mother's behavior whereas the implicit assumption in research prior to that time had been that the caretaker's behavior caused the behavior of the child. Others have extended the research on reciprocal caretaker-child behavior to include secondary caretakers, primarily teachers. Thomas and Chess (1977) have found compelling clinical evidence which suggests that the temperament characteristics of a child may strongly influence a teacher's perceptions and expectations of that child.

Korn (1977) reports the results of a correlational study relating temperament characteristics to reading and arithmetic achievement scores. In this study low academic achievement scores were significantly associated with the behavioral dimensions characteristic of the "Slow-to-Warm-Up" child, adaptability and approach. In addition, Seegars (1977) found that teachers tended to underestimate the intellectual capabilities of the "Slow-to-Warm-Up" child. It was hypothesized that the expectations of the teachers may have influenced the actual learning that subsequently occurred. Gordon and Thomas (1967) also demonstrated that the qualities of adaptability and approach affected teachers' judgments of children's intelligence. In another study (Carey, Fox, and McDevitt, 1977) it again was found that children's adaptability was significantly correlated with teacher perceptions of children's adjustment to school.

Another area in which temperament research may have direct practical significance to educators is that of special education. In a recent study, Carey, McDevitt and Baker (1979) compared temperament profiles of normal children with temperament profiles of children in four other diagnostic groups: minimal brain dysfunction (MBD), hyperactivity, learning disability and other (generally emotional disturbance). Many of these "problem" children had been referred to the pediatric neurologist by teachers and other school personnel.

The results demonstrated that those children diagnosed as "problems" differed significantly from normal children on four characteristics: lower adaptability, lower persistence, higher activity levels and lower approach. This "problem" group also was disproportionately represented in the "Difficult" child category.

The children in the MBD group differed from normal children on four variables: lower adaptability, lower persistence, higher activity level, and more negative mood. Children in the hyperactive and learning-disabled group were similarly low in adaptability and persistence. Those children in the fourth diagnostic category differed from normal children on three variables: lower adaptability, lower persistence and higher activity level.

Of the "problem" children referred to the neurologist, all were distinguished from normal children at least by lower adaptability. However, only about half were found to have objective neurological signs. The researchers suggest that the referring teachers often mistook differences in behavioral *style* for behavioral *problems* with neurological origins.

It appears that a teacher's perceptions of a child's behavioral style in the school setting can strongly influence important judgments about that child. A child's general rate of adaptability seems to be the recurring variable that teachers perceive as indicative of a child's adjustment. How the teachers interpret a child's adaptability level appears to influence their judgments not only about general adjustment to school, but about intellectual capabilities of the child. Most importantly, adaptability level appears to affect teachers' evaluations of the "normality" and "abnormality" of the student. These judgments, in turn can have an enormous impact on the child's self-regard.

Perhaps the development of the Teacher Temperament Questionnaire (Thomas and Chess, 1977) is a positive initial step in recognizing teachers as an important part of the temperament-environment interactive process. Its use may help to develop an appreciation of individual differences in behavioral style on the part of professional educators. Carey (1979, 1981) suggests that consideration be given to including a temperament assessment not only in the diagnostic procedures for potential special children, but also in the evaluation procedures for school adjustment problems and academic achievement difficulties. Just as we have accepted the notions of widely varying maturation rates, and intellectual developmental differences, so must we begin to accept that behavioral style dimensions are an important source of individual differences.

REFERENCE NOTES

1. Fullard, W., McDevitt, S. C., and Carey, W. B. Toddler Temperament Scale, 1978, Unpublished test form, available from William Fullard, Ph.D., Dept. of Educational Psychology, Temple University, Philadelphia, PA 19122. Please send $5.00 to cover costs.

2. Hegvik, R., McDevitt, S. C., and Carey, W. B. Middle Childhood Temperament Questionnaire, 1980, Unpublished test form, available from Ms. Robin Hegvik, 307 North Wayne Ave., Wayne, PA 19087. Please send $5.00 to cover costs.

REFERENCES

Bell, Richard Q. A reinterpretation of the direction of effects in the studies of socialization. *Psychological Review*, 1968, *75*, 2; 81-95.

Buss, A. H. and Plomin, R. A. *A temperament theory of personality development*. New York: Wiley-Interscience, 1975.

Carey, W. B. A simplified method for measuring infant temperament. *Journal of Pediatrics*, 1970, *77*, 188-194.

Carey, W. B. The importance of temperament-environment interaction for child health and development. In M. Lewis and L. Rosenblum (Eds.), *The uncommon child*. New York: Plenum Press, 1981.

Carey, W.B., Fox, M., and McDevitt, S. Temperament as a factor in early school adjustment. *Pediatrics*, 1977, *60*, 621-624.

Carey W. B., and McDevitt, S. Revision of the infant temperament questionnaire. *Pediatrics*, 1978, *61*, 735-739.

Carey, W.B., McDevitt, S., and Baker, D. Differentiating minimal brain dysfunction and temperament. *Development Medicine and Child Neurology*, 1979, *21*, 765-772.

Gordon, E.M., and Thomas, A. Children's behavioral style and the teacher's appraisal of their intelligence. *Journal of School Psychology*, 1967, *5*, 292-300.

McDevitt, S., and Carey, W. B. The measurement of temperament in 3-7 year old children. *Journal of Child Psychology and Psychiatry*, 1978, *19*, 245-253.

Rowe, D., and Plomin, R. Temperament in early childhood. *Journal of Personality Assessment*, 1977, *41*, 150-156.

Thomas, A., and Chess, S. *Temperament and development*. New York: Brunner/Mazel, 1977.

Thomas, A., Chess, S., and Birch, H. G. The origin of personality. *Scientific American*, 1970, *223*, 10-2-109.

Thomas, A., Chess, S., Birch, H. G., Hertzig, M. E., and Korn, S. *Behavioral individuality in childhood*. New York: New York University Press, 1963.

DRAMATIC PLAY AS A DIAGNOSTIC AID IN THE PRESCHOOL

Nancy E. Curry, PhD
Sara H. Arnaud, PhD

ABSTRACT. Dramatic play, if facilitated by adults, is a universal phenomenon in young children. Deviance from the developmental trends of play suggests the need for diagnosis, which is possible only if there are ample opportunities for dramatic play in the classroom. An overview is given of developmental trends in the play of three, four, and five year olds with emphasis on their themes, modes, and social interactions, and discussion of warning signs in those areas. Since the meaning of play behavior is multiply determined, readers are encouraged to use observation of dramatic play as one important piece in the total picture of the puzzling child.

As the teacher surveys the tapestry of free play in her four-year group, she notices children playing together in a large block building they have constructed with sleeping spaces outlined for each one, a well equipped kitchen and a garage full of "missiles" ready to launch. They have labeled their building "No aliens allowed" and have devised an elaborate ticket system for admission to the "missile factory." Molly, in her Wonder Woman Underroos, is flashing her magic bracelet and imperiously ordering three followers to do her bid-

Address inquiries to: Nancy E. Curry, PhD, Professor and Program Director, Program in Child Development and Child Care, School of Health Related Professions, University of Pittsburgh, Pittsburgh, PA 15261, or Sarah H. Arnaud, PhD, Professor of Psychology, Program in Child Development and Child Care, School of Health Related Professions, University of Pittsburgh, Pittsburgh, PA 15261.

ding. One child challenges her authority. Molly hesitates, then capitulates by proposing a solution in which each of them gets something he or she wants. The teacher smiles to herself in appreciation of how Molly's accommodations have succeeded in keeping all the children involved in and enjoying their play.

Why then does the same teacher inwardly groan when she turns and sees Tommy sitting on the radiator cover, a Batman cape draped around his shoulders pretending to drive a Batmobile to no particular destination, just as he has been doing every morning for the past three months? When another child comes by and announces he is Batman too, Tommy angrily retorts, "Get out of here! *I* am Batman!" For three months he has played this and no other role, with an intensity that obliterates his ability to join in other play and even in mundane daily routines like snack. Tommy's mother too has complained that this type of play dominates activities at home. Although the thematic content of Tommy's play, like Molly's, is superheroes, there is a quantitative and qualitative difference in the way the theme is elaborated, how others are involved, and the richness of the character and plot they enact.

The questions this paper will attempt to address are the ones teachers and parents often pose:

—What is appropriate dramatic play?
—When does dramatic play signal underlying difficulties?
—What might individual children's play tell us that would help in diagnosis for remedial action or indicate the advisability of referral for other professional help?

Universality of Play in Young Children

For young children, play is the most natural and spontaneous of activities, on a par with eating, sleeping, motility and elimination. Of the many sorts of play indulged in by preschoolers, we will concentrate on dramatic play. The content and mode of dramatic play show strong developmental trends. Anything that is deviant in this natural development of dramatic play deserves scrutiny.

Before the teacher can use play as a diagnostic tool, however, it is essential that he or she ensures that there is ample opportunity for depthful play in an environment that encourages and facilitates self-expression through play, and where less than happy and less than pleasant play themes are tolerated (Arnaud & Curry, 1974). The example of superhero play was deliberately introduced because it is of almost universal interest to children and yet many parents and teachers become so uncomfortable with it that they stop it even before it starts. The very themes that are the most likely to produce intense investment in children are the ones most likely to make many adults uneasy. The still "uncivilized" impulses of childhood produce discomfort in all of us: children pretending they are poisoning another unsuspecting child, fights to the death between animals, playing monster.

Overview of Developmental Trends in Dramatic Play

Given a benign, facilitating environment, most three year olds will have developed the capacity to symbolize their internal and external experiences through simple dramatic play. These symbolizations become more elaborate with age, and occur in the following areas:

—What the child chooses to symbolize—the theme
—How the child symbolizes—mode
—And with whom—social interactions

These give us a powerful lens to examine children's self-representations—how they see and feel about themselves. Careful examination of a young child's dramatic play provides a potent diagnostic aid for assessing health and pathology in physical, emotional, cognitive, and social development.

Below is a brief recapitulation of the developmental sequences in dramatic play proposed in earlier work (Arnaud & Curry, 1973; Curry & Arnaud, 1974), which can provide a normative baseline for evaluating the play of preschoolers.

Three Year Olds

Themes. Three year olds' themes vary from transparent imitation of daily scenes to occasional incursions into frightening fantasy. While placid domestic themes dominate, with nurturance and caretaking as a central focus (good mommies, helpful doctors), one also sees wild animals, monsters, and superheroes—themes in which the aggression is unmodulated or at the most, thinly veiled. Parents may come across these normal but frightening fantasies more often than teachers, in the child's fear of darkness, imagined ferocious animals in closet or under bed, and bad dreams.

Mode. The play of the three year old has a fragmentary feel to it, as the child attends to the aspect of a role that has the greatest current salience for him or her (e.g., the stethescope around the neck designates that she is playing doctor, while the actual doctoring activities are minimal). Further, roles seem fluid and shift easily and quickly (the erstwhile doctor plops into a cradle and deposes the bemused "patient").

Being rather than *pretending to be* the portrayed character is to be expected for two year olds and early three year olds. In fact, distinguishing between reality and pretend is a major task at this age, with many three year olds displaying what Gould (1973) calls "fluctuating certainty"—that is, a child may start pretending to be a tiger and suddenly become overwhelmed by aggressive affect to the point of actually acting out the tiger who bites and scratches and hurts. As children make the necessary cognitive oscillations between accommodation (imitation) and assimilation (play), they are concurrently advancing affectively from the introjection of the meaningful persons in their lives, to identification with them.

Additionally, later threes are able to describe their activities (I'm playing racing cars) which show an awareness of themselves as agents and generators of play plots.

Social interactions. One expects some social interaction with peers in the play of three year olds, especially where common interests surface and require reciprocity (mother/baby, doctor/parent, zoo keeper/animals). Mutual developmental concerns will spark parallel play (bathing babies, bedtime preparations, meal preparation); but cooperative play still taxes the cognitive and social capacities of most three year olds.

Four Year Olds

Themes. Developmental pressures seem to mount in the four year old. Thematic content of play shifts in balance from the more bucolic themes of the threes to heightened struggles around aggression. While caretaking roles continue, dramatic play themes are elaborated to include more role aspects (e.g., firefighters eat at the firehouse, rescue people, and put out fires to the accompaniment of siren sounds and much rushing around).

By this age, self-representation in play also embraces a wider range of play characters, indicating the child's recognition of the array of role possibilities in the world outside the home (service professionals, ghosts, witches, monsters, folk heroes, fairytale characters, prehistoric animals, etc.). Gould's (1973) concept of the behavioral clusters that coalesce around primary identification of nurturant provider, aggressor, and victim are useful at this stage. A child's inability to move comfortably and flexibly between these identification is a cause for concern and further study.

Mode. Four year olds demonstrate a capacity for "distance from self" in their moving from self-action (e.g., playing they are fire fighters) to toy-action through the use of miniature life toys (Arnaud & Curry, 1973)—e.g., in addition to dressing up in the accoutrements of a fire fighter, a child may also use the small rubber figures to enact the drama of rescuing children from a burning school.

Their ability to maintain the distinction between real and pretend should now be well established, with the expectation that play will be used to sublimate raw emotions into socially acceptable and useful channels.

Social interactions. Four year olds are somewhat fickle social beings, who nevertheless have the ability to engage in cooperative play if the theme taps into their current developmental preoccupations. Yet enduring friendships among peers are common; inclusion is so important that they will exclude others in order to assure themselves that they are included.

Five Year Olds

Themes. By this age children have the capacity to play out most aspects of the world as they know and experience it, as well as aspects they have not yet concretely experienced but are trying to understand (weddings, husband and wife roles). Adult activities are subjected to children's close scrutiny and provide nutriment for many depthful play episodes. Five year olds attempt to master their fears of the many unknowns by personifying them in dramatic play (e.g., having a ghost arrive to rouse and terrify peaceably sleeping children; setting up a "haunted house" as part of an elaborate block structure).

Mode. Building on the three year old's direct representation of a role and the toy-action one sees at four, five year olds will devise rudimentary scenarios even more distant from self, such as puppet shows and simple plays. Their play episodes will have a discernible beginning, middle, and end; they will show foresight and planning.

Social interactions. Cooperative play abounds at five, with children making skillful accommodations to each other in order to sustain a gripping play idea. Feelings continue to run high, but five year olds have the ability and desire to compromise. Friendships are intense; at this age, children are more likely to try to please each other so they can remain part of a group, than they are to woo adults.

Warning Signs and Significant Patterns

It is dangerous to interpret a child's play in the light of one instance or one sample. This paper attempts to put into behavioral terms what it is about the child's cues that stirs the observer's uneasiness. We are emphatically not concerned with quick and easy diagnosis.

A specific pattern of overt behavior may arise from any one of a number of possible sources. Diagnosis and/or causation usually must be determined by examining many facets of the child's experience: through consideration of developmental history, parental attitudes and behaviors, stresses in the home, physical health, reactions to standardized procedures such as psychological tests, neurological examinations, etc.

Thematic Content

Easily observable deviations can be picked up when themes are clearly inappropriate for the child's age. For instance, intense, realistic, absorbing baby play is to be expected at three but not at five. When a five year old insists on enacting such a role for long periods of time, he/she may do so for a variety of reasons: attempting to master the fact of once again being displaced by the birth of a new sibling; or because the cognitive demands of the kindergarten are beyond the child's intellectual capabilities (with other evidence such as delayed speech, difficulty with puzzles, poor social skills, abnormal physical movements, etc.); or being overwhelmed by a recent trauma such as hospitalization or an accident; or totally shutting out the stimulation of a classroom because of an inability to sort out diverse stimuli in the more discriminating fashion of other age mates.

A child who is singlemindedly preoccupied with one theme or one role (e.g., victim) over time alerts the caregiver to the fact that expected flexibility and variety in play have been interrupted. Day after day, five-year-old Pauline could not seem to lure the other children to her endless unelaborated and prosaic mother-baby play. Instead the playmates she sought were busily performing "heart transplants," building kennels for a family of circus dogs and creating other diverting dramas. Pauline's clinging to her early themes and inability to fathom her age mates' more complicated play was one of the early clues to her mild retardation.

While we expect most children to work at resolving traumatic events through re-enacting them in play, occasionally a child will be caught up in a repetitive re-enactment that brings no relief or mastery. The play of the kidnapped children of Chowchilla (Terr, 1979) is an example of such fruitless play.

Highly unusual play themes are also worth studying. They may only reflect a vivid, unusual experience that the child is trying to master—that is, be based on reality rather than fantasy. It turned out that four-year-old Chuck who repeatedly herded imaginary people into an enclosure while saying threateningly, "Put 'em in the tank," had actually been temporarily put in a jail cell with the rest of his family after their driver was stopped for reckless, drunken driving. Without a reality base for such unusual play, one needs to take a close look at what is propelling the play.

Experiences of molestation and/or other abuse may surface in veiled play that has a furtive, driven quality. Four-year-old Claire would intersperse her generally unelaborated house play with giggling references to "bum bums" and tense excitement around having dolls kiss and undress. Further, she would urgently and anxiously plead with unsuspecting male staff members to kiss her or to go into enclosed spaces where they could be alone. Subsequently, her mother confirmed that there had been overt sexual activity between Claire and a grandparent.

Excessive preoccupation with ordinary objects that assume highly symbolic and idiosyncratic significance (e.g., trains, garbage cans, record players, shampoo) may be indicative of more severe psychopathological processes, as is bizarre fantasy content revealed in dramatic play (e.g., a child who became terrified playing outdoors in the sunshine because "the sun is stealing my power").

Mode of Dramatic Play

The play of young children often has a sober, workmanlike quality, just as there may be light-hearted, even giddy, hilarious moments. But play that has a driven intensity raises a warning flag for caregivers. When play stops being a choice for the child and appears obligatory and compulsive, we know the child is responding to impelling internal pressures and/or preoccupations.

Excessive rigidity in dramatic play may be another harbinger of severe emotional difficulties or a response to overwhelming external pressures (so that the child attempts to hold himself together through inflexible efforts to control his play world), or it may reflect a lack of cognitive skills to expand play beyond the stereotyped known.

Children whose play is fluid, fleeting, and fragmentary deserve a closer look to determine if they are incapable of a higher level of play (developmentally delayed), if they do not have the ability to sort out pertinent stimuli and thus respond equally and indiscriminately to any available stimuli (nervous system impairment), or if they are preoccupied with internal imagery which intrudes on their capacity to perceive reality clearly (emotional disturbance), or if an acute or chronic trauma is absorbing too much energy for them to be able to cope with their current play world.

One should be concerned if children are not able to take a distance from the role they enact, and instead, under the guise of play, launch aggressive attacks in which they *are* rather than pretend to be the aggressor (the unleashed tornado, the biting monster, the rampaging elephant). Aggression for such children tends to be annihilative, rather than competitive (Speers & Morter, 1980). They both fear and provoke it in others, whose intentions they assume to be as hostile as their own. Once again, one needs corroborative evidence to determine whether such aggressive outbursts are reactions to environmental pressures, including the frustrations children feel if they are unable to cope physically, intellectually, or emotionally with external circumstances, or are expressions of internal pressures which the child lacks the ego capacities to control.

Social Interactions in Dramatic Play

Older preschoolers who cannot tolerate the intrusion of other children in their play, who actively seek solitude, or who seem completely oblivious to other children, bear watching. Again, it is the quality of the interaction or non-interaction that may serve as a diagnostic sign. Developmentally delayed children may have the social skills of much younger children which include short attention span, inability to see another child's point of view or to follow an elaborate play idea. Children with attention disorders may prefer to play on their own because of their tendency to become disorganized under the impact of too much stimulation from other children. The content of play of disturbed children may be so private that they choose to isolate themselves in rapt engrossment with their fantasies.

Some children prefer the presence of other children, but cannot sustain productive interaction. It is important to note when and how the interaction breaks down. A child whose aggression is raw and unmodulated may be ever on the alert for suspected attacks from other children and "hit back first." Lack of cognitive awareness, with its resultant bemusement and/or obliviousness about what is going on in a complex play sequence, may cause a child to blunder into and disrupt on-going play. If such a child is physically or mentally handicapped, he may join a play episode and in the frustration of not being able to follow the plot or action, lash out and spoil it for the others as well.

Caregivers should be alert to the children who cannot play on their own, who are compelled to seek out other children (often a specific admired child), as alter ego, in a twinning fashion. These children seem to lack a solid sense of self, and feel the need for the continuous support of another child. Only when one intervenes in such twinning behavior and observes the child in situations where he or she has to operate without another child, can one determine what deficit the child is attempting to make up through leaning on the stronger child.

The social behavior of other children toward a given child is often revealing. Children who are consistently avoided, scapegoated, or actively rejected usually provoke these reactions in their peers. Abused children, for example, seem to perpetuate their victim status by inciting verbal or physical abuse from other children. The behavior of impulse-driven youngsters can be terrifying to adults and children alike, but children are more likely to act on their fears of the unpredictable by avoiding or rejecting such a child in their play.

Summary

All of us have worked with children whose behavior both troubles and puzzles us. We are recommending that caregivers consider the dramatic play of young children as a key piece in the total behavioral picture of individual children. Their play tells us a great deal about their developmental status, individual concerns, capabilities, weaknesses, strengths, and social maturity.

When you see marked and persistent deviation from usual developmental trends in dramatic play, look at it carefully, then look again to see if it occurs only in certain specific circumstances. Then ask someone else to look at it with you—through in-house consultation or referral to other professionals for further exploration. The results of a multi-focussed diagnostic assessment will help you determine whether the problem can be dealt with in the current setting or whether it merits referral to an appropriate service agency (such as child guidance center, developmental clinic, special school).

REFERENCES

Arnaud, S. H., & Curry, N. E. (Producers). *Role enactment in children's play: A developmental overview*. New York: Campus Film Distributors, 1973. (Film)

Arnaud, S. H., & Curry, N. E. (Producers). *The facilitation of children's dramatic play*. New York: Campus Film Distributors, 1974. (Film)

Curry, N. E., & Arnaud, S. H. Cognitive implications of children's spontaneous role play. *Theory into practice*, 1974, *13*, 273-277.

Gould, R. *Child studies through fantasy*. New York: Quadrangle Books, 1973.

Speers, R. W., & Morter, D. C. Overindividuation and underseparation in the pseudo mature child. In R. Lax, S. Back & A. Burland (Eds.), *Rapprochement*. New York: Jason Aronson, 1980.

Terr, L. C. Children on Chowchilla: A study of psychic trauma. In A.J. Solnit, R.S. Eissler et al. (Eds.) *Psychoanalytic study of the child* (Vol. 34). New York: International Universities Press, 1979.

INTERPRETING CHILDREN'S PLAY

Anthony D. Pellegrini, PhD

ABSTRACT. This paper discusses categories by which puzzling children can be identified by observing their play. Categories for interpreting children's play are outlined for cognitive play, social play, and play with language. Descriptors of normative behavior for each of these modes of play are provided. Recommendations for further assessment are made for each play mode.

The intent of this paper is to provide a framework by which observers can make inferences about identifying puzzling children and their development by observing children's play. More specifically, systems for categorizing children's play along cognitive, social, and linguistic continua will be described. Interpretations, based on the current psychological literature, for each form of play exhibited will be discussed. These interpretations may indicate a child's need of more observation and possibly referred for further assessment.

Play has been defined as a process whereby children assimilate new experiences into pre-existing cognitive structures (Piaget, 1962), that is, children familiarize themselves with new objects and people by interacting with them in a goal-free and pleasurable situation (Garvey, 1977). For example, children who have never encountered an inflated balloon can familiarize themselves with the properties comprising this object by playing with the balloon. Such play would be characterized by the children applying actions and concepts they have already mastered to learn about the balloon. They may roll and bounce it

Anthony D. Pellegrini is in the Early Childhood Education Department, 427 Aderhold Hall, University of Georgia, Athens, GA 30602.

because it resembles a familiar beach ball. Through such playful interaction children acquire the concept of a balloon as being a round, bouncing object.

Cognitive Aspects of Play

Developmental psychologists (Piaget, 1962; Fein, 1979) have suggested that insight into children's cognitive ability can be gained by observing children's pretend play. Smilansky (1968) has developed a system, based on Piaget (1962), which enables an observer to categorize children's play along a cognitive hierarchy. This hierarchy has been empirically verified by Rubin and Maioni (1975) and Pellegrini (1980). It consists of four categories: functional, constructive, sociodramatic play, and games-with-rules. Functional play precedes, developmentally, the other forms of play.

Functional Play

Functional play is characteristic of the period 0-1½ years of age. It has the children simply exercising their muscles (with or without objects), e.g., squeezing a ball, babbling, pounding the floor. A hallmark of functional play is repetitious movement. For example, infants can be observed often repeating the same sound or continually splashing water. Functional play enables the children to explore objects in their environments and the effect their actions have on the environment. Through functional play children practice those actions that are needed for higher forms of play. *If by 1½ years children have not mastered simple motor exercises system, e.g., hand-eye coordination, babbling freely, locomotion by crawling, further diagnosis may be required.*

Constructive Play

The next stage of cognitive play developmentally observed is constructive play. In constructive play the child works towards a goal, e.g., building a tower, drawing a picture, or building with blocks. Children from about 1½-3 years of age should be capable of using the actions and materials used in functional play for the play themes characteristic of constructive play. *If by 3-3½ years of age, children's free play actions are not theme- or construction-oriented, the children's cognitive strategies and motor skills should be more closely diagnosed.*

Sociodramatic Play

The third stage of cognitive play is sociodramatic play. In this form of play, children use language to take on fantasy roles, e.g., playing house, cowboys, or dress-up. Children between 3-6 years of age typically engage in sociodramatic play. Smilansky has listed five criteria children must meet in order to do sociodramatic play. First, children must imitate another's role. Children of this age often imitate adult roles such as mother or father. Secondly, children should engage in make-believe with regard to objects. For example, a child may have a broom represent a guitar. As children grow older, the objects they use as props to represent other objects become more abstract. For example, three year olds may need a broom to represent a guitar whereas six year olds would not use a prop at all to represent a guitar. They may use their hands to strum on an invisible instrument. The third criterion has children sustaining their play for at least ten minutes. Fourth, more than one child must be involved in the play episode. Fifth, children must use oral language in the play episodes. Language should be used to tell players the roles props can represent and to define players' roles.

If children by the age of six years are not capable of meeting all of these criteria, play intervention strategies may be necessary. Smilansky (1971) has outlined specific strategies for facilitating children's sociodramatic play. Smilansky (1971) outlined a program adults can use to help young children meet each criterion. In this model adults intervene into play episodes as players to facilitate play.

Games-with-Rules

The highest form of cognitive play, play according to Smilansky (1968) and Piaget (1962), is games-with-rules. Children do not typically engage in games-with-rules until 7-11 years of age because of the complex cognitive processes involved in such a mode of play. Games-with-rules are governed by rules established by others. In lower forms of play children establish their own rules of play, e.g., have a desk and chair represent an automobile. Games-with-rules have children subordinating their actions to an externally imposed set of rules. For example, if a child is called out on strikes in a baseball game, he/she must give-up his/her turn at bat.

Thus, through observing children playing games-with-rules we can determine the extent to which they are willing and able to obey arbitrary rules. Failure to follow rules may be a cognitive problem, e.g., not able to comprehend or remember the rules, or a social problem, e.g., not willing to share in the rules established by others.

Social Aspects of Play

Parten (1932) has outlined a system to interpret the social play of children. Just as the cognitive aspect of children's play seems to develop hierarchically so too does the social aspect of play. Infants' social play, 0-1 year of age, is often *unoccupied behavior.*

Unoccupied Behavior

This type of play has the infant in a social setting not engaging in any form of action. For example, an infant may be observing puppets interact. Prolonged periods of unoccupied behavior may indicate that children are wary of exploring their environments. Children of this age should normally spend much time exploring their environment. Such behavior in a social context typifies the child until 2½ years of age. These children comprehend the notion that other people exist but they do not possess the social skills necessary to initiate and sustain social interaction. Therefore, adults should not be alarmed when children of this age do not initiate or readily respond to social interaction.

Solitary Play

Forms of solitary play include playing with puzzles or mobiles, solitary animal talk. Unoccupied and solitary play are typical behaviors for children 0-2½ years of age. *If children do not progress socially after this age period, concern is warranted. Children of this age should spend their time exploring their physical environment. Gradually they should want to explore social relations.*

Parallel Play

Parallel play marks the beginning of social interaction. Children 3-4 years old often play next to other playing children and use similar materials but do not interact with them. Children engaged in projects such as painting and drawing are good examples of parallel play. Parallel play is often observed in house-keeping corners. Two young girls may both be playing "mother" in the same play kitchen but not interact with one another. Children engaged in parallel play *are aware* of the other children's presence but they do not possess the social skills necessary to initiate play. Adults should encourage the parallel play of 3-4 year olds by complementing the parallel players on becoming playmates.

Associative Play

Associative play is the next stage of social play. Associative play is characteristic of children approximately 3½-4½ years of age. Associative play has children playing at a common activity where materials and interests are shared. Children building one block structure together, not two separate structures, is a good example of associative play. Players in associative play, however, do not remain constant. The specific group composition of children building a structure with blocks, will continually change as children leave and join the group at will. Children of this age do not subordinate individual interests to the interests of a group.

Cooperative Play

The highest form of social play is cooperative play. Cooperative play is not usually observed until the child is older than 4½ years. Children in cooperative play are organized as a group for the purpose of a common goal. Examples of cooperative play include sociodramatic play, hop-scotch, and group projects.

The age norms for social play provided by Parten suggest that children younger than 3 years of age should not be expected to sustain social interaction with peers or adults. However, this age child should soon begin to show an interest in other persons. Parallel playing is the first sign of the ability to engage in social play. Children, as they develop the necessary social skills, will become more adept at initiating and sustaining play. We must remember that children from infancy (Garvey, 1977) are interested in other people. They need help in developing the skills needed to sustain this interaction and considering others' points of view. Adults should not expect children to be *adept at these skills*. Adults can encourage social play by having children play with objects in the vicinity of other children as adults. Solitary play with objects should progress to more social forms of play, ie., parallel and associative.

Rating the Complexity of Play

These social and cognitive models have been used to rate children's developmental status. The age range corresponding to each of the cognitive and social descriptors provides a normative reference point. Secondly, the hierarchic nature of each system would lead one to infer about the complexity of children's play. For example, a child doing dramatic play would be viewed as being cognitively more advanced than an age-mate doing constructive play. Similarly in the social arena, children engaging in associative play are seen as more mature than children engaging in parallel play. For these reasons researchers (Rubin, 1977; Sponseller & Jaworski, 1979) have used these categories to construct matrices whereby children's cognitive and social play can be categorized and interpreted.

More specifically, a child's single play episode can be categorized simultaneously along cognitive and social dimensions. Using these dimensions the social and cognitive complexity of children's play can be ranked. Because both cognitive and social schemes are hierarchic, i.e., lower forms of play are less complex than higher forms, we can assign a rank to each form of play. Within the cognitive scheme functional play is least complex so it is given a rank of 1. Constructive play, rank 2, is more complex than functional but less complex than sociodramatic play (3). Games-with-rules are most complex and ranked 4. A similar ranking system can be used for social play. Unoccupied play is least complex so it gets a rank of 1, followed by solitary (2), parallel (3), associative (4), and cooperative play (5). A play complexity score is derived, first, by categorizing the social *and* cognitive aspects of one play episode. The rank score for the social dimension should be multiplied by the cognitive rank. The resulting product is the complexity score. For example, Sue is painting along at an easel next to John. Cognitively, Sue is engaged in constructive play because her play is theme oriented; her cognitive rank is 2. Socially, because

Figure 1

Play Complexity Matrix*

	Cognitive			
Social	Functional$_1$	Constructive$_2$	Dramatic$_3$	Games - Rules$_4$
Onlooking 1 Solitary 2 Parallel 3 Associative 4 Cooperative 5				

*Based on model used by Rubin & Maioni, 1975.

she is playing next to John, she is categorized as doing parallel play, ranked 3. Her play complexity rank of 6, is derived by multiplying her social rank of 3 (parallel play) times the cognitive rank of 2 (constructive). A rank of 20, then, is normal for a six year old. Such a system should be used to chart the growth of individual child play. Weekly records should be kept of each child's play complexity. *If one child is not progressing at the same rate as others, closer attention or diagnosis may be needed.* It should be noted that this system of analyzing children's social and cognitive play is only one of many forms of diagnosis. Other forms, such as diagnostic tests, should be used to complement this system.

Speech Play

The next aspect of play to be examined is children's play with language, or speech play. Speech play has the speaker manipulating the phonological, syntactic, and semantic aspects of language with little concern for the traditional goal of language use: conveying a message to a listener.

Through the process of playfully manipulating the aspects of language young children gain a knowledge of the linguistic rule system. For example, through a word substitution game such as:

—The stove is hot
—The pot is hot
—The water is hot

children are manipulating words in one grammatical, or syntactic category; a class of nouns which can be used in a syntactic subject.

Children's awareness of the rules of their linguistic system has been labelled as metalinguistic awareness (Cazden, 1974; Chomsky, 1979). Metalinguistic awareness is often an end product of speech play because in play episodes, the rule system of language itself is manipulated. Speech play, then, like other forms of play, is a mode whereby young children explore and manipulate the many aspects of their language system. Metalinguistic awareness is the end product of speech play. Examples of metalinguistic awareness include children's awareness that certain words are not phonologically possible in English, e.g., *TDIS*, or that certain sentences are not syntactically possible, e.g., *The slow is here*.

Researchers have found that children play with aspects of language in hierarchical order (Kirshenblatt-Gimblet, 1976); that is children tend to play with sound, or phonological, aspects before the grammatic, syntactic, meaning, or semantic aspects of language. In this section each aspect of play will be discussed separately in the order in which each appears.

Phonology

Children first play with phonology, or the sound system of language (Garvey, 1977). During the babbling period, from birth to ten months of age, infants explore all the sounds in the human linguistic system. Gradually, they limit sound play to only the sounds of their native language (DeStefano, 1978). These repetitive and rhythmic vocalizations are usually generated when prelinguistic children are in pleasurable states. During this time they learn the "shape" of their language by experimenting with stress and intonation patterns present in the language they here. Such speech play is characterized by chanting sequences of nonsense syllables which have the same stress and intonation patterns as words in their native language. This type of speech play is typically generated by children to accompany their solitary play actions.

Thus for the first two years of life children's speech play is typified by babbling in solitary and social settings. *Children by the end of this period should be practicing the sounds native to their language. If the child is unable to articulate certain sounds, further diagnosis should be considered.*

Play with phonology for children two years of age and older takes place in the presence of adults or other children, i.e., social contexts. The social phonological play of two year olds is exemplified by use of conventional noises, through syllable repetition, to identify actions, events, and objects, e.g., *ruff-ruff, vroom*. Thus, the phonological play of children older than two years should be social. Two children may be playing parallel or associatively with trucks. Their phonological play would be the *vroom* sound of truck engines.

Syntax and Semantics

Play with phonology continues through adulthood, though, by two years of age children should begin playing with other aspects of language. At approximately two to three years of age children have been observed playing with the syntax and semantics of language (Garvey, 1977; Weir, 1962). Knowledge of syntax, or how words are ordered in utterances to convey meaning, is gained when children manipulate whole sentences or syntactic elements within sentences. For example, children have been observed changing declarative sentences into interrogatives, e.g., *It's here. Is it here*? In such cases children learn about syntactic transformations. Weir's son, Anthony, manipulated whole sentences through reduction/expansion techniques, e.g., *Here it is. Here it is now. Here.* Anthony also explored acceptable words for individual syntactic categories through word substitution games, e.g., *He runs fast. He swims fast.* Noun to pronoun substitutions were also observed, e.g., *John is here. He's here. Who's here*?

Word replacement games also have a semantic (meaning) dimension. Weir found that Anthony's replacement games differed qualitatively from games of older children and adults. Anthony's first word placement games consisted of using words which were syntagmatically related, e.g., *The mat is here. The cat is here.* Syntagmatic classifications are based on superficial perceptual associations, such as phonetic rhymes. Syntagmatic pairs often occur together in children's speech or physical environments. Older children's replacements tend to be conceptually, or paradigmatically, related, e.g., *The pin is here. The needle is here.* Conceptual groupings consist of words from the same conceptual category. This qualitative shift from syntagmatic to conceptual grouping reflects the different conceptual systems of younger and older children. Ability to use words that are conceptually related in word replacement games is a result of children's general cognitive development.

Given this relationship, observers can use the word play generated by children to gain insight into children's cognitive processes. For example, if children's semantic word play does not group conceptually related words (conceptual grouping) they may not be able to group items conceptually. They may only be capable of grouping items which they observe together (syntagmatic groupings). Like phonological play, play with syntax and semantics continues through adulthood. We can use play with syntax and semantics to chart children's linguistic skills (Pellegrini, 1981). As children develop they should play with words paradigmatically. Their syntactic play should involve longer sentences and many different types of transformations. For example, they should change declaratives to questions, imperatives, and exclamatives, not only declarative to questions.

This paper has attempted to provide a framework to categorize children's play. It is hoped that the systems presented here will be used by persons in the helping professions to gain insight in children's developmental status. We believe that play provides a valid means of assessing children's cognitive, social and linguistic competence. Figure 2 summarizes these interpretations of play.

Figure 2

Summary of interpretive play categories by age*

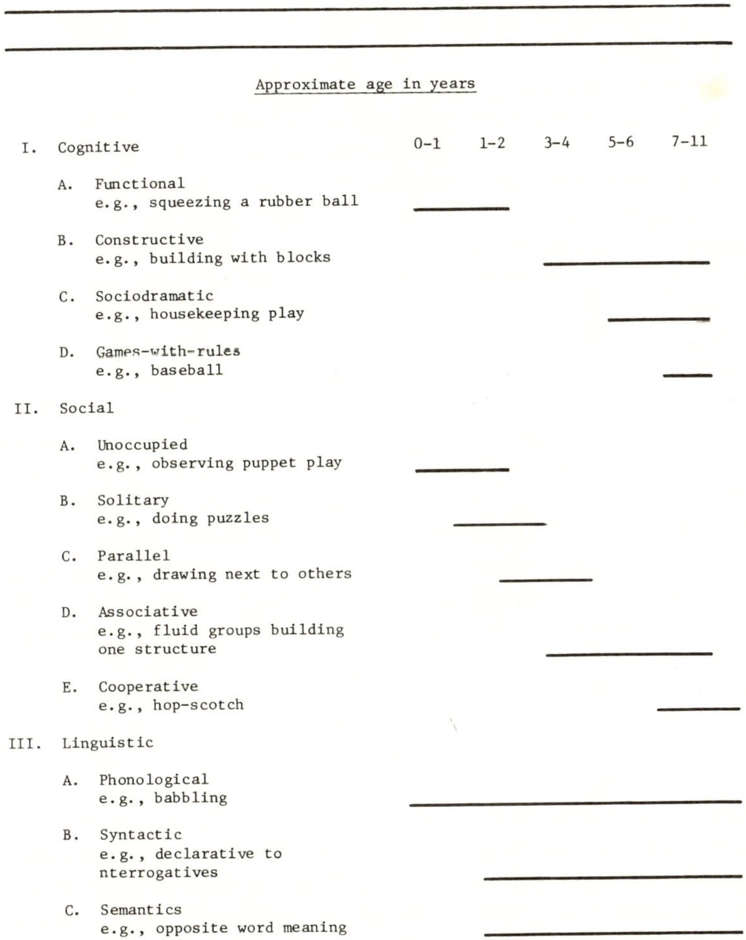

*Based on models by Rubin & Maioni (1975) and Pellegrini (1981)

REFERENCES

Chomsky, C. Consciousness is relevant to linguistic awareness. Paper presented at International Reading Association Seminar on Linguistic Awareness and Learning to Read, June 1979, Victoria, British Columbia.

DeStefano, J. *Language, the learner, and the school*. New York: Wiley, 1978.

Fein, G. Plan and the acquisition of symbols. In L. Katz (Ed.), *Current Topics in early childhood education, Volume II*. Norwood, New Jersey: Ablex, 1979.

Garvey, C. *Play*. Cambridge: Harvard, 1977.

Jakobson, R. Linguistics and poetics. In T. Sebeok (Ed.), *Style in language*. Cambridge: MIT Press, 1960.

Kirshenblatt-Gimblet, B. (Ed.). *Speech play*, Philadelphia: University of Pennsylvania Press, 1976.

Parten, M. Social participation among preschool children. *Journal of Abnormal Psychology*, 1932, *27*, 243-269.

Piaget, J. *Play, dreams, and imitation*. New York: Norton, 1962.

Pellegrini, A. The relationship between kindergartners' play and achievement in prereading, language, and writing. *Psychology in the Schools*, 1980, *17*, 530-535.

Pellegrini, A. Speech play and language development. *Journal of Research and Development in Education,* 1981, *14,* 73-80.

Rubin, K. The play behaviors of young children. *Young Children*, 1977, *32*, 16-24.

Rubin, K., & Maioni, T. L. Play preference and its relationship to egocentricism, popularity and classification skills in preschoolers. *Merrill-Palmer Quarterly*, 1975, *21*, 171-179.

Smilansky, S. *The effects of sociodramatic play on disadvantaged preschool children*. New York: Wiley, 1968.

Smilansky, S. Can adults facilitate play? In N. Curry, & S. Arnaud, (Eds.), *Play*. Washington, D.C.: NAEYC, 1971, 39-50.

Sponseller, D., & Jaworski, A. Social and cognitive complexity in young children's play. Paper presented at the Annual Meeting of the AERA, April 1979, San Francisco.

Weir, R. *Language in the crib*. The Hague: Mouton, 1962.

INTERPRETING THE BEHAVIORS OF CHILDREN

Craig B. Liden, MD
Theresa E. Laurie, PhD
Timothy F. Murphy, PhD

ABSTRACT. Estimates indicate that large numbers of children (4-20%) experience developmental problems which affect their learning and/or behavior. Understanding and interpreting the behaviors such children present, is a challenging and difficult task. Our current unidisciplinary procedures for assessment and intervention frequently result in narrow or inaccurate explanations for the child's behavior. Comprehensive assessment procedures are needed which can uncover all of the complex factors (biological/physical, emotional, cognitive, and environmental) which contribute to the developmental problems of children. In this article the authors outline the philosophy and procedures for a comprehensive, transdisciplinary approach to interpreting the behaviors of children and intervening to resolve learning and behavior problems. This approach described is currently being used and researched at the Child Development Unit of Children's Hospital in Pittsburgh, Pennsylvania.

Dr. Liden is Assistant Professor of Pediatrics at the University of Pittsburgh and Director of the Child Development Unit at Children's Hospital of Pittsburgh. Dr. Laurie is an Assistant Professor of Pediatrics and Special Education at University of Pittsburgh and Educational Program Coordinator of the Child Development Unit at Children's Hospital of Pittsburgh, and Dr. Murphy is Assistant Professor of Pediatrics at University of Pittsburgh and Developmental Psychologist at the Child Development Unit, Children's Hospital of Pittsburgh. Requests for reprints should be addressed to Craig B. Liden, MD, Children's Hospital of Pittsburgh, 125 DeSoto Street, Pittsburgh, PA 15213.

The authors acknowledge the contributions of William I. Cohen, MD, and Kathleen Connolloy, MSW, and the efforts of Carol Hallberg in preparing the manuscript.

Introduction

Tommy Jones is five years old and is having problems, "He fights with his brother and sister, frequently breaks his toys, and doesn't sleep well at night." Since Tommy entered kindergarten, things have gotten worse. His teacher indicates that, "Tommy is out of his seat, doesn't finish work, and has fights with other children."

The kindergarten teacher wonders what is wrong with Tommy and his parents. She expressed her anguish to his mother by stating that, "Tommy is extremely immature, and perhaps he is not ready for kindergarten." Mrs. Jones is concerned that Tommy's problems in school may be related to her new job and the marital problems she and her husband are experiencing.

In an attempt to understand Tommy's behavior, Mrs. Jones sought help from various professionals. Each interpreted Tommy's behavior differently:

Tommy's pediatrician saw him and determined from the health, birth records, and the physical examination that everything was *normal.* He patted Mrs. Jones on the hand to reassure her that Tommy was "all boy and will grow out of it." (Mrs. Jones wondered how she will make it until Tommy changes.)

The school social worker viewed Tommy's behavior as a reaction to stresses in his family. The Jones's were encouraged to spend more time with Tommy, and to seek counselling. (Mrs. Jones felt guilty about her new job.)

The school psychologist evaluated Tommy and determined that he had a learning disability and recommended that Tommy be placed in the Perceptual Kindergarten. (Mrs. Jones wondered what this meant and if she had done anything to cause the problem.)

At the end of her experiences, Mrs. Jones was even more confused about Tommy's behavior. She still wondered what to do about it. Like the blind men who described the elephant by touching the part nearest to them, each professional had focused only on one aspect of the situation. Operating in isolation from one another, disciplinary biases determined their explanations, while none provided a comprehensive interpretation to adequately address Tommy's problems in the home and in the school.

The experiences of Mrs. Jones are re-enacted daily as parent, teachers, and professionals seek to understand and address the problems of many young children. Estimates indicate that subtle developmental disorders affect 4-20% (Minskoff, 1973) of the children in our country. Interpreting the behaviors of young children like Tommy is an extremely difficult task for professionals. The problems in our current approaches to assessment and intervention with young children have long been recognized and the need for more comprehensive models which can define the reciprocal interactions between children and their environment has been identified (Brindley and Bell, 1981; Deneberg, 1979; Sameroff and Chandler, 1975). Unfortunately, few models for such approaches exist, and most professionals in the field have not been exposed to broader, multidisciplinary assessment practices. To be a service to children and families, assessment procedures must be used which address the complex nature of such subtle developmental disorders. In this paper, a multidisciplinary and comprehensive approach to address such problems will be described. Such an approach is an alternative to the unidisciplinary methods used by professionals like those consulted by Mrs. Jones.

Philosophical Basis for a Multidisciplinary Approach to Assessment and Intervention

The strategies to be described are based upon some important underlying premises:

I. There are a multitude of factors, both environmental and constitutional that are known to or are suggested to influence development, learning, and/or behavioral potential in a given child. The number of these factors that influence life "performance is constantly increasing as a child develops chronologically."

II. There is a "continuum of causality" (Sameroff and Chandler, 1975) with respect to the outcome of developmental risk factors, such as those mentioned above. These factors do not necessarily impact on an individual child in an "all or none" fashion. The variability within and between children suggests that individual children may respond differentially to the same risk factors.

III. A child's functional status at any point in time is the product of a series of *transactions* between constitutional factors (intrinsic qualities) and environmental factors and life events. The majority of developmental or behavioral dysfunctions are *not* simply the result of the *unidimensional* progression of a *single* risk factor that can be ascertained through a process of "ruling out" medical and social factors. Rather, these dysfunctions more often are the result of reciprocal interactions between certain constitutional and environmental risk factors over time that are unique for each child. Therefore, a successful diagnostic and therapeutic approach to developmental dysfunctions must include not only a comprehensive exploration of constitutional and environmental risk factors but an attempt to understand transactions between them. "Etiology," and therefore successful "treatment," more often becomes apparent through an understanding of these reciprocal interactions than through extensive, and often poorly thought through and expensive, diagnostic studies geared to rule out all possibilities.

IV. Risk factors may demonstrate a differential impact on developmental and behavioral outcome as a function of *time* (in terms of age) of occurrence. That is, an insult may have radically different effects on developmental outcome if it occurs at age three months versus the same insult occurring at 12 months. Furthermore, clear cut manifestations of a given insult may require variable amounts of time to display themselves.

V. *Dysfunction* is a term used to describe performance failure which cannot be attributed exclusively to a specific etiology. Most performance failure in childhood falls within this category.

VI. Dysfunction in childhood is the product of constitutional predispositions of a child that have transacted with environmental influences. The intrinsic predispositions may be present at birth but often only manifest themselves when the environment requires efficient performance.

VII. A major developmental challenge for children and parents involves the acceptance of the predispositions intrinsic to a child. This is particularly true with respect to developmental functions underlying efficient learning, social interaction, and behavioral organization. For these functions, early signs are not necessarily overt but rather subtle and difficult to identify.

VIII. The mismatching or inappropriate environmental responsiveness (expectations) to constitutional predispositions and individuality may be a major mechanism leading to manifest dysfunction. Therefore, early description of a child may lead to valuable guidance and the prevention or minimization of dysfunction. This primarily involves bringing environmental expectations in accord with a child's emerging pattern of strengths and weaknesses.

IX. There is a commonality to the behavioral manifestations of a wide variety of developmental dysfunctions.

Summary

The goal and purpose of the assessment and intervention strategies based upon these premises is the generation of a comprehensive description of the child and the environment. Such a description can lead to a deeper understanding of the current problem. To insure that the assessment procedures result in a *better* understanding of the child's behavior, the professional's activities must be guided by the following questions:

—What new, disordered or unrealistic expectations are being set for this child?
—What factors in the environment (past and current, home and school) may be contributing to the problem?
—What is the child's current level of functioning in all areas: physical, cognitive, emotional?
—How do all the factors (within the child and the environment) interact together to provide an explanation of the current problem?

A Common Diagnostic Process

By synthesizing current knowledge about the basic principles of child development and the characteristics of learning and behavioral dysfunction, it is possible to define a comprehensive common diagnostic process that can be applied to presenting problems from infancy through adolescence. Such a process is schematically presented in Figure 1. In order to address the complexities of problems like Tommy's, this process requires the participation of representatives

FIGURE 1

THE COMMON DIAGNOSTIC PROCESS

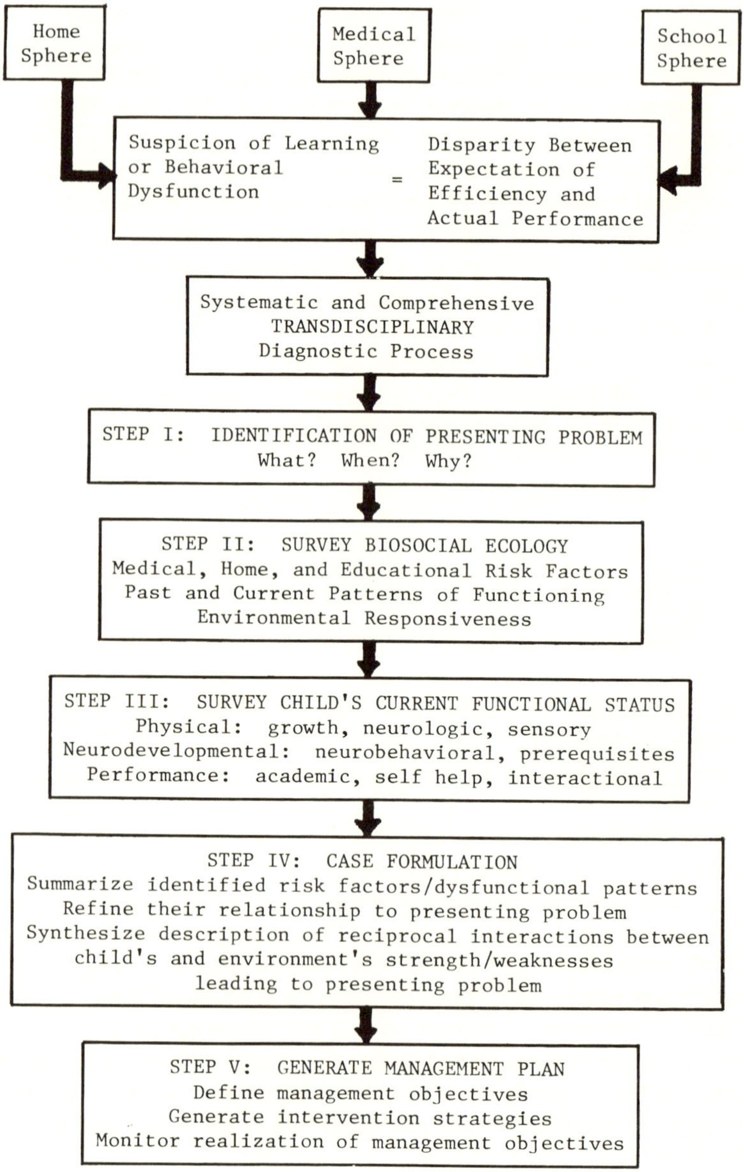

from a variety of disciplines including education, pediatrics, social work, psychology, and speech pathology among others. Furthermore, it is necessary for these professionals to move beyond their disciplinary boundaries and to function as "transdisciplinaries" so that they can understand how the diverse factors intrinsic to the child and those present in the environment *reciprocally interact* to lead to the learning or behavioral dysfunctions. This transdisciplinary approach facilitates the establishment of an efficient and effective diagnostic-therapeutic continuum where assessment findings can readily and meaningfully be translated into an intervention plan. This is unlike many multidisciplinary approaches in which professionals execute their part of the process in isolation and simply tabulate their findings without synthesizing them into a comprehensive description of the problem and plan of action.

The following is an overview of the steps involved in implementing this Common Diagnostic Process. Objectives and the clinical activity involved for each step are summarized.

STEP 1 - Identifying the Presenting Problem

> *Objective*: To clearly identify and define the parameters of the presenting problem.
>
> *Clinical Activity*: Initial interview with referral source.

As was stated previously, it is critical for the clinician to have a precise understanding of the problem behavior. Since a problem must be viewed as a symptom of the child not meeting the environment's expectations for performance, great care must be taken to learn what it is the child is or isn't doing and what the adult thinks the child *should* be doing (i.e., the *expected behavior*).

It is also important to learn how the adults are currently explaining or interpreting the child's behavior. Their interpretation is an indication of the attitudes and beliefs they have formed as a result of their own thinking or from information they have obtained from relatives, neighbors, *other professionals*, etc. If this information is put out in the open, it can be used directly when the clinician provides his/her explanation for the problem. The current belief may need to be altered (through the sharing of new evidence) before the adult can accept a new or different interpretation of the problem.

In order to clearly identify and bind the presenting problem in this fashion, the initial interview with the referral source (most commonly the parents) should *always* include the following questions:

1. In your own words, what are your *specific* concerns about this child?
2. When did you *first* develop these concerns?
3. What made you seek help for this problem *at this time*?
4. What do you think may be *causing* this problem?
5. Do you have any *fears* about this problem?
6. Before now, what have you done to manage this problem?
7. What do you expect can be done about this problem?

STEP 2 - Survey the Biosocial Ecology of the Problem

Objectives: To identify factors in the medical, home and school spheres that may have impacted on the child or his environment in such a fashion as to contribute to the presenting problem.

To identify patterns of functioning which may be intrinsic to the child and the environments response to these patterns which may have contributed to the genesis of the presenting problem.

To identify parental (and school) perceptions of the child's current physical, neurodevelopmental, and performance strengths and weaknesses.

Clinical Activities: Completion of Parent and School Questionnaires; Review of Previous Data (Medical records, school records, previous testing, etc.); Extended Parent Interview (Psychosocial).

Through questionnaires, actual records or extended interview, historical information is collected about the child. This information is not necessarily gathered to identify *a* causal factor, but rather to learn about *significant* events which *may* have impacted on the child or the environment, and to gather a perspective regarding the child's past and current patterns of functioning. This can be accomplished by systematically surveying the child's medical, home and school experiences for the presence of the following risk factors:

Medical Sphere:

1. *Pregnancy, Perinatal, and Early Health Risk Factors*: Although retrospective research has indicated that these risk factors appear to occur with a high frequency in the histories of children with learning and behavior problems, it is not clear why. Prospective studies suggest that this is *not* a simple cause/effect relationship. (Sameroff and Chandler, 1975).
2. *Somatic Dysfunctions*: Children with learning and behavior problems show a higher incidence of problems such as enuresis (wetting), encopresis (soiling), headaches, etc.
3. *Delayed Developmental Milestones*: Frequently, children attain these gross markers of "normal" development at age appropriate or accelerated intervals. When this occurs, parents are frequently confused and find it difficult to understand how this "normally" developing child can be experiencing difficulty.
4. *Temperamental Dsyfunction*: The literature has suggested that the child's temperamental style, activity level, rhythmicity, distractibility, sensitivity to and reaction to changes, attention span and mood are relatively stable from infancy to adult life (Chess and Thomas, 1971). When a child demonstrates extremes in these intrinsic characteristics, they may interfere with efficient interactions with the environment.
5. *Familial Risk Factors*: There is some evidence to suggest that learning and behavioral problems show a familial tendency. It is unclear whether this reflects a genetic inheritance or propagation of dysfunctional learning and behavior patterns through parental reinforcement.

Home Sphere:

Information is also gathered about the following:

1. *Disordered Parental Expectations*: The parents' current expectations for the child need to be defined to uncover the current performance demands for the child.
2. *Management/Discipline Difficulties*: Frequently, parents of children with developmental problems experience great difficulty setting and keeping limits for behavior. These problems

may be due to the child's intrinsic characteristics being at odds with parents' methods.

3. *Insufficient Support Systems*: The presence of children with unique learning and behavioral needs in a family, oftentimes creates a need for support for the parents (good friends, family). More, the absence of such a network may exacerbate the situation by the parents being alone and unsupported through difficult times they encounter.
4. *Life Stress Events*: Certainly, stressful events in the life of the child or family may contribute to the current situation (divorce, death, financial difficulty). Especially, if the child is susceptible to such stresses due to his/her sensitivity and temperamental profile.
5. *Peer Relationship Difficulties*: Children with delayed functioning or temperamental and attentional problems frequently experience difficulty establishing or maintaining age appropriate relationships.
6. *Diminished Self-Esteem*: Even in the early years, children with developmental problems may lack confidence in their abilities due to a history of failure and negative feedback from the adults in their environment.

School Sphere:

1. *Historical Educational Performance Failure*: Oftentimes children have had a chronic history of failure of difficulty in a school setting. However, on occasion the problem may appear to be sudden as a result of novel demands being placed upon the child.
2. *Disordered Educational Expectations*: The school's current requirements for the child are defined to clarify the disparate expectations which are contributing to the problem.
3. *Insufficient Program Resources*: Frequently children may be difficult for the school to handle given limits in economics, program and material resources. The support available needs to be defined to help determine what might be encountered in seeking additional support in the school.
4. *Management/Discipline Difficulties*: Developmentally delayed children frequently create difficulties in a classroom. The nature

of these difficulties and the current methods for management need to be defined.

Information gathered about risk factors should be supplemented by a survey of the parents' (and teachers) perceptions about the child's *current* functional status in the following areas:

—Physical
—Temperamental/Attentional
—Developmental
—Social Interactional
—Academic
—Self-Help (Independent Functioning)

This information can be useful to increase the reliability of and to help focus the clinician's direct assessment of the child (Step 3) and to identify disparity between parents', teachers, or the clinician's perceptions about the child's current functioning that may help explain an aspect of the presenting problem.

STEP 3 - Survey the Child's Current Functional Status

Objectives: To identify abnormal physical findings in the child that may contribute to the presenting problem.

To identify inefficient neurodevelopmental functions that may contribute to the presenting problem.

To identify inefficient performance skills that may contribute to the presenting problem.

Clinical Activities: Physical Assessment; Neurodevelopmental Assessment; Educational Assessment; Child Interview-Behavioral Observations.

Physical Assessment: Many purely medical conditions may manifest themselves in dysfunctional behavioral patterns, therefore, a complete assessment of the child's current health status is necessary. The physical assessment includes identification of abnormal findings in:

1. Growth
2. General Physical Factors

3. Gross Neurological Function
4. Sensory Function
5. Morphogenesis

Neurodevelopmental Assessment: Information should be collected on a variety of subtle neurological and developmental factors that underlie efficient learning and behavior. This assessment should include identification of inefficient functioning in the following areas:

1. *Neurobehavioral Functions*:

   (a) *Neuromaturation* - The underlying neurological maturity and organization of the child can be evaluated through the presence or absence of so-called "soft signs", primitive reflexes and efficiency of gross motor function. Neuromaturation is not presumed to bear a direct relationship to academic or behavioral performance, but is seen as a possible indicator of factors intrinsic to the child which may signal dysfunctions in Central Nervous System (CNS) development. In this sense, neuromaturation is viewed as a measure of the "soil" in which other skills develop.
   (b) *Attention* - The assessment of attentional efficiency should be done in the context of a structured task. It includes observations of the child's cognitive tempo (balance between impulsivity and reflectivity), ability to filter out distractions and focus on a task, vigilance or attention span and monitoring skills or ability to critically evaluate the accuracy of his/her performance.
   (c) *Temperament* - Parent and teacher perceptions of temperament can be supplemented by the clinician's observations of these stylistic characteristics during the course of the evaluation.

2. *Prerequisite Functions*: During the neurodevelopmental examination, information should also be collected on the child's ability to receive, integrate, and respond to information. A child's unique pattern of processing information can be determined through direct assessment of inefficiencies in the following areas:

   (a) *Auditory Sequential Memory*: listening to and remembering a sequence of spoken information.

(b) *Visual Sequential Memory*: watching and remembering a sequence of visual information.
(c) *Receptive Language*: understanding spoken language (single words and connected speech).
(d) *Expressive Language*: using spoken language, appropriate vocabulary and syntax (including articulation).
(e) *Fine Motor/Visual Motor Integration*: using small muscles of the hand in coordinated fashion to draw or write.
(f) *Higher Order Cognitive Functions*: classifying and categorizing information; understanding part/whole relationships; using problem solving abilities; drawing conclusions, generalizing, and rules.

A comprehensive neurodevelopmental assessment can help provide understanding the child's unique pattern of strengths and weaknesses.

3. *Educational Assessment*: Each child's skill in the area of preacademic and academic skills must be surveyed to determine what skills he/she has acquired. Depending upon the child's age, information is collected on inefficiencies in the following areas:

   1. *Readiness*: Knowledge of colors, shapes, letters and numerals, discrimination, recognition of, names of.
   2. *Language Arts*: More elaborate listening skills, and expressive language skills.
   3. *Reading*: Knowledge of letter/sound relationships, sight vocabulary, decoding, oral reading, and comprehension.
   4. *Spelling*: Knowledge of spelling patterns, rules for adding endings.
   5. *Math*: Counting skills, number concepts, more advanced knowledge of number concepts, and concepts of time, money measurements, place value, and computation.

The child's current academic functioning can be defined to the curricular demands of preschool or school, and specific understandings of the child's individual needs and abilities will emerge.

Child Interview/Behavioral Observations: During the course of the direct assessment of the child, the clinician should systematically look for inefficiencies or inappropriate behaviors in the following areas:

1. *Cooperativeness*: The ease with which the child worked together with evaluators to complete tasks.
2. *Response to Reinforcement*: The degree to which praise or disapproval resulted in a change in child's behavior.
3. *Affect*: The degree to which the child's disposition matched the circumstances of the evaluation.
4. *Thought Process*: The degree to which the child's ideas logically follow one another.
5. *Self-Esteem*: How the child appeared to feel about him/herself.

Demonstrated weaknesses in these behavioral areas not only may contribute to an understanding of the presenting problem, but along with inefficiencies in attention, and extremes in temperament, may also adversely impact on the child's performance on various neurodevelopmental and educational tasks administered during the assessment. Unless behavioral inefficiencies are taken into account, the clinician may get an inaccurate picture of the child's current functional status in these prerequisite and performance areas.

It is important to note that while Step 3 has stressed identification of weaknesses or inefficiencies, it is equally important for the clinician to conduct a comprehensive assessment that allows for detection of areas of strength as well. Mobilizing such strengths can be an important part of a comprehensive management plan.

STEP 4 - Case Formulation

Objectives: To systematically categorize the identified biosocial risk factors, the child's inefficient physical, neurodevelopmental, and educational functions, and the child's and environment's past and current patterns of functioning generated in Step 2 and 3.

To refine the relationship of the risk factors, inefficient skills and patterns of functioning to each other and to the presenting problem.

To generate a synthesized description of the child's and the environment's strengths and weaknesses and their hypothesized interactions that may relate to the presenting problem.

Clinical Activity: Transdisciplinary Staffing

After all the historical or current information is collected about the child and the child's environment, this information must be carefully formulated into a descriptive understanding. This is most efficiently done by conducting a *staffing conference* including all the professionals who have been involved in the evaluation. The primary responsible clinician on the team should gather evaluation data from the other professionals involved in order to have an objective summary of:

1. The child's strengths and weaknesses in all domains of functioning (past and current).
2. The Home and School environments' strengths and weaknesses (past and current).

Once this information is summarized, the team must then begin the process of refining the potential relationship of environment risk factors and inefficiencies in the child's current physical, neurodevelopmental, and performance status to the presenting problem. With respect to environmental risk factors, the team may ask the following questions to help them decide if these factors *contribute* to the presenting problem:

—Has the risk factor altered an aspect of the child's constitutional development in such a fashion as to result in a functional weakness that directly contributes to an aspect of the presenting problem?

—Has the risk factor altered the environment's expectations or perceptions of the child in such a fashion as to impact on it's (the environment's) interactions with the child resulting in either the emergence of other risk factors and/or physical, neurobehavioral, prerequisite, or performance inefficiencies or abnormalities that directly contribute to an aspect of the presenting problem?

—Has the risk factors been demonstrated in the literature or through clinical experience to be a frequent early manifestation of either the presenting problem itself, another risk factor directly associated with the presenting problem or a physical, neurobehavioral, prerequisite or performance inefficiency or abnormality associated with the presenting problem?

—Has the risk factor been demonstrated in the literature or through clinical experience to frequently occur jointly or concurrently with either the presenting problem itself, another risk factor directly associated with the presenting problem, or a physical, neurobehavioral, prerequisite or performance inefficiency or abnormality associated with the presenting problem?

An affirmative answer to one or more of these questions clearly suggests a decision that the risk factor is contributory to the presenting problem.

With respect to identified physical, neurodevelopmental or performance inefficiencies, the team again must decide whether these factors contribute to the presenting problem. In making this decision, they must ask the following question:

> Is the identified inefficiency a necessary prerequisite for the *expected behavior* (i.e., the behavior which the child is failing to demonstrate as manifest by the presenting problem), or a component part of that behavior.

Again an affirmative answer to this question suggests that the inefficiency is contributory to the presenting problem.

In turn, the contributory biosocial risk factors and inefficient skills are integrated into a comprehensive description of the presenting problem (Case Formulation). This can be accomplished by a synthesis of how the child's weaknesses are mismatched with the conditions and demands in his home and school environments, and by clarifying the transactions that may be occurring. With this comprehensive analysis comes a more accurate plan to deal with the problem. In general, the efficacy of a treatment plan is dependent upon the adequacy of this synthesized description.

STEP 5 - Generating and Implementing a Plan of Action

> *Objective*: To utilize the case formulation for *definition* of specific objectives for management of the presenting problem.
>
> To generate specific intervention strategies for each of the management objectives.
>
> To monitor treatment efficacy by longitudinally assessing realization of management objectives.

Clinical Activities: Transdisciplinary Staffing; Parent/Referral Source Conference; Follow-up.

In implementing a plan of action, it is critical to share the explanation or interpretation of the problem behaviors with the referring adult. In answering initial questions or clarifying concerns, the clinician must carefully and clearly describe the factors within the child and the environment which appear to be contributing to the problem. The adult will need to assimilate this new awareness into his/her belief system for real understanding to occur. The professional needs a structure to insure that this renewed understanding can be translated into appropriate actions to improve the current situation. To do this, objectives and strategies are generated to address all of the factors which have been judged as contributory to the problem. This includes the following:

1. Oftentimes the assessment raises the need for additional information. An objective and a plan of action is developed to acquire the needed information.
2. Certainly one of the first objectives to accomplish in any case is to help the adults in the child's environment *reorder or modify their current* expectations for their child. The professional helps translate the parents' understanding to specific inappropriate expectations. For the problems to be alleviated, the environmental demands must be more closely matched to the child's unique pattern of functioning. The more accurate expectations may be translated to the environment's acceptance of the child and the provision of necessary emotional, material, personal, or structural supports to improve the child's functioning.
3. Some of the management plans need to be targeted to the contributory factors within the child. This may take the form of medical interventions when necessary, or specific *remedial or compensatory* strategies to address the child's intrinsic weaknesses or inefficiencies. For each factor within the child and the environment, specific objectives and plans are developed. Specific plans to reach these objectives must be developed with the involvement of the child's parent or teacher to increase the likelihood of implementation. The implementation of these plans should be monitored longitudinally by the coordinating professional in the form of follow-up visits. Objective informa-

tion can be collected from the parent, the teacher, to assess progress. Actual re-evaluation of the child, if repeated, can help to document progress. As time passes, frequently the management plans must be altered to address new events, occurrences, or the frequency of interaction with the family is reduced or even terminated. Such extensive management plans which attempt to "hit on all fronts" are more likely to result in progress.

Conclusion

Perhaps if Mrs. Jones had had access to such an evaluation her experiences in understanding and interpreting Tommy's behavior could have been avoided.

Comprehensive assessment and intervention procedures are necessary to adequately interpret and address the behaviors of children with developmental disorders. Such complex problems are always a result of multiple factors intrinsic to the child and within the environment. Therefore intervention procedures must involve a variety of disciplines so all aspects of the problem can be understood. The result of such assessment procedures is a broad understanding of the problem, and not simplistic interpretations which may be inaccurate due to limited information on only one aspect of the problem. Professionals working with such young children have an important opportunity to prevent children from later failure, and to help them maximize their potential. Through the use of a comprehensive approach to early intervention, professionals will be more likely to reach these goals.

REFERENCES

Brindley, S., and Bell, R. Issues in early identification. In Kaufmann, J. and Hallahan, D. (eds.), *Handbook of special education*, New Jersey: Prentice-Hall, 1981.

Chess, S., and Thomas, A. *Temperament and development*, New York: Brunner-Mazel, 1977.

Denenberg, V. H. Dilemmas and Designs for Developmental Research. In C. L. Ludlow and M. E. Diran-Quine (eds.), *The neurological basis of language disorders in children: Methods and directors for research,* NINCDS Monographs, Washington, DC: Government Printing Office, 1979.

Minskoff, J. G. Differential approach to prevalence estimates of learning disabilities. *Annual New York Academy of Science*, 1973, *205*:139.

Sameroff, A., and Chandler, M. Reproductive risk and the continuum of caretaking causalty. In Horowitz, F. (ed.), *Review of child development research*, Vol. 4, Chicago: Chicago University Press, 1975.

INTERVENING IN CHILD'S PLAY

Thomas Daniels Yawkey
Susan Louise Trostle

Overview

The use of intervention and guidance by adults who guide young children at play is not new to early childhood (Singer, 1973; Axline, 1947). The new twists characteristic of current approaches to play intervention emphasize the importance of imaginative play to children's intellectual (as well as social/emotional) growth. These new twists and contemporary views rest on a number of research-supported assumptions concerning the importance of intervention and imaginative play in young children.

First, play—specifically pretend, imaginative or make-believe play—is defined as the children's ability to change themselves into

Thomas Yawkey is an Associate Professor of Early Childhood Education, Early Childhood Faculty, Division of Curriculum and Instruction, The Pennsylvania State University, University Park, PA and President, Pennsylvania Association for Childhood Education. Susan Trostle is a Graduate Assistant in the Early Childhood Program Speciality and teaches courses in Children's Literature in the Division of Curriculum and Instruction, The Pennsylvania State University, University Park, PA.

The senior author gratefully acknowledges financial support from the Research and Program Development Division, The Economy Company Educational Publishers, Oklahoma City, Oklahoma; The Pennsylvania State University's College of Education Alumni Society Research Fund, University Park, Pennsylvania; and The Margaret M. Patton Foundation, Kittanning, Pennsylvania for providing research funds for investigations upon which portions of this narrative are based.

other individuals, situations, and events as observed through their verbal and/or motoric actions (Curry & Arnaud, 1974). In this sense, imaginative play is viewed as a necessary ingredient of intellectual growth (Piaget, 1962). Playing "Wonder Woman," "Daddy," "cat," "tree" or "Tooth Fairy" requires the youngster to view himself "as if" he is another. The mental capacity to image in "as if" form links imaginative play with intellectual processes. Second, play, and especially make-believe play for children from low income populations, is often underdeveloped (Smilansky, 1968). Differences between children in their use of imaginative play can be explained by variations in the quality and quantity of play things found in the youngsters' environment.

Third, imaginative play actions and activities can be constructively shaped, reinforced and trained in varying degrees:

a. through manipulation of the quality and quantity of play materials in the child's environment;
b. by increasing the opportunities for youngsters to use and show play;
c. through teachers and parents suggestions aimed at encouraging playful interactions between youngsters and their play environments (Yawkey & Fox, 1981)

Results from several studies show that guiding children in playing fairy tales such as "Three Little Pigs" and "Three Billy Goats Gruff" and in playing prior experiences, for example, "Going Shopping in East Mall" and "Visiting the Circus" encourage significantly their imagination, playfulness, and intellectual abilities. In addition, through adult guidance in imaginative play, oral language growth for these children improves substantially (Pellegrini, 1980).

Linking play to intellectual growth takes on new dimensions in contemporary approaches to intervention in child's play in school and home. The push for return to play in early childhood and the dynamic utility of play intervention strategies provide the basic keys to other significant dimensions of young children's intellectual and social/emotional growth for teachers and parents.

Play Intervention: Some Approaches and Strategies

Play intervention can make sound contributions to the young child's imaginative, intellectual, social/emotional and language growth. Given the importance of play intervention to development, children of all ages can benefit from its use. In working with and intervening in children's play, teachers and parents approach children with aims of observing and interpreting it and then employing selective strategies to encourage and facilitate playing actions and activities. By observing and interpreting children's play as baseline criteria for intervening in play routines, teachers and parents can follow and use the relevant suggestions proposed by Curry, Arnaud and Pellegrini on interpreting play in their respective articles in this issue. For example, the helpful model for the dimensions of social play as proposed by Parten (1932) suggests that play unfolds along a continuum from onlooker or unoccupied to solitary, parallel, associative, and cooperative play.

Briefly, play at the onlooker level is characterized by children's watching the actions and activities of others, objects, and situations. Solitary play is characterized by children's verbal and/or motor play with themselves; the attributes of parallel play are individual and personal motor and/or verbal involvement of children with no genuine social interaction. The youngsters may be sitting side-by-side or in group settings. Associative play is characterized by children interacting with each other at low and superficial levels of interaction. Last, play at the cooperative level is characterized by meaningful communication between children who plan, define and assign their play roles and proceed to carry them out in social group settings.

Unioning Parten's approach, which gives a baseline for observing and interpreting play routines of young children, with selected strategies used by adults to encourage the levels of play, a usable intervention model is possible. The strategies that can be employed by teachers and parents to intervene in, and thereby encourage, solitary, parallel, associative, and cooperative child's play are: (a) time and space; (b) adult guidance; (c) play materials; (d) boundaries; and, (e) roles played.

The first strategy, time and space, asks teachers and parents to provide time in the daily schedule and enough space in the environment for children to play. The second strategy, called adult guidance, requires teachers and parents to sensitively offer oral language prompts as they play (e.g., "I wonder if baby wants some milk to drink!") and direct involvement cues (e.g., "That was really delicious!" says Mrs. Mack as she pretends to eat the ubiquitous birthday cake). Play materials, the third strategy, focuses on providing a variety of play materials for youngsters to use in their play. For example, making materials available from each of the categories of constructional (e.g., blocks, tinkertoys, lincoln logs), instructional (e.g., nesting cubes, puzzles), real materials (e.g., sand, water, navy beans, wood) and toys (e.g., trucks, dolls) gives variety and provides the children with opportunities to choose those that they want to use in their play routines.

The fourth strategy that teachers and parents use to intervene in children's play is boundaries. In using this strategy of boundaries, adults show youngsters, through demonstration and practice, how to enter and leave play situations. Play is facilitated as youngsters enter group play routines, perhaps by observing and easing into them, rather than by breaking into the routines and demanding, "I want to play!" The final strategy, roles played, asks teachers and parents to let the youngsters decide upon their own play themes and define and assign their roles. Adults can also, at times, suggest some play themes for specific instructional purposes. In addition, this strategy focuses on children rotating roles in the play episode, playing it again and making sure that all of them have the opportunity to participate.

Using Parten's approach to observe and interpret play behaviors and the five teacher and parent strategies for facilitating play provides a complete intervention model for use with young children playing in a variety of ways. The following section gives examples of using this intervention approach and strategies in school and home settings.

Play Intervention: Some Examples

The following examples, which illustrate intervention strategies, require teachers and parents to observe and interpret the level at which the youngsters are playing. Effectively using the strategies with them at that level is the natural, resultant outcome of observing and interpreting.

Onlooker Play

Watching others play can become a stimulating developmental and learning experience. First, the youngster decides for himself which play group, action or activity he wants to observe. Then, using the time and space strategy, the youngster may decide to spend five to eight minutes or longer watching one or more activities in varying settings. To accommodate the onlooker as well as the player, particular areas of the classroom are allotted to play routines of the youngsters.

Although the requirements of space depend on type and kind of onlooker play, designing particular play areas of the classroom as play areas reinforces the importance of the child's play. Here, it is important to remember that the time and space used appropriately in onlooker play stimulates the child to play creatively on his own.

Second, in using the strategy of adult guidance, the alert teacher or parent keeps one eye upon the onlooker and the other on the players. Onlooker's reactions to: (a) conversation; (b) objects; (c) actions; and (d) themes in the play episode provide valuable clues about the youngster's areas of interest and familiarity. The adult's questions, comments and enthusiastic responses encourage the onlooker and player to sustain interest in the play. For instance, the child smiles broadly and chuckles while watching two peers as they "roll" make-believe apples and bananas from play dough and pretend to nibble on them. In guiding the onlooker, you can focus his attention on particular aspects of the pretend by saying, for example, "Bobby and Jema are pretending to eat the tasty fruit. Doesn't it taste delicious!" Or, the onlooker may cover his eyes while the Cookie Monster puppet attacks thc Ernic puppet. You could comment, "I wonder how Ernie feels!" Guidance encourages the onlooker to think about particular aspects of the play he is observing and maximizes the potential for him to join the play routines. The third intervention strategy is the use of play materials. In onlooker play, the youngster watches a set of blocks being used in a variety of ways, for example. A block becomes a truck, charging down the freeway. Later, the onlooker notes that the block is a frog, sitting on a lillypad. Seeing many new uses for familiar toys, and conversely discovering that many toys can represent familiar themes, the youngster sees one object substituted for another. Careful, perceptive listening and observing of the youngster, while in the onlooker and in other daily-occurring roles and situations, informs the caretaker as to the youngster's readiness for watching and using different play materials.

Boundaries, the entering and leaving of play situations, is the fourth strategy. Its use varies widely with the age of the onlooker. Some will enter and leave the play setting; others will remain for longer periods of time and perhaps even join the players. Boundaries for the onlooker should remain flexible so that the child may come and go as he pleases.

The final strategy for use with the onlooker concerns the roles played by the participants. In the interest of the onlooker, as well as the players, variety in both language and visual experiences is heightened when the young players rotate roles and inject fresh themes. Although the participant's ideas remain foremost, the adult nonetheless suggests a variation upon a theme or character portrayal at times. For instance, youngsters flying to the moon can, in addition, fly to Mars or around the world.

Solitary Play

The time and space strategy for the solitary player is an important school and home consideration. The child's rate of intellectual growth is enhanced through provision of a regular, daily scheduled time for play. The solitary player becomes engrossed with his individual exploration and personal arrangement of the toys. Solitary players require time to understand their play routines as they enact them. The size of the space for solitary players is determined by the child's play themes and areas of interest. When the room is partitioned into separate play areas (for example, large muscle, housekeeping or instructional toys), the child is encouraged and reinforced for playing accordingly in each area.

Using the guidance strategy as the solitary player, for example, progresses from the toy dishes to the pirate ship and costume corner to the painting area, the adult's role is mainly one of attentive observation. Reflecting the child's play themes and transitions, as well as the emotions and statements portrayed, you encourage and motivate the child at play. While the youngster climbs on the top step, holding a twisted coat hanger and shouting, "I'll find the buried treasure!", you use the guidance strategy by saying, for example, "I wonder where Captain Hook can hunt for the treasure!" Careful and accurate reflections of the child's play themes and verbalizations are necessary; occasional summary or intent statements are in order for the guidance strategy to be effectively used in solitary play. You can say for instance, "You're really interested in pirates and ships today. You're excited about the story of Peter Pan we heard (or saw on TV)!" Stepping beyond the simple reflective mode, you can also use modeling and within-role suggestions as guidance strategies for the solitary player. For example, you can hold up a Miss Piggy puppet as the child manipulates Kermit the Frog. You squeak, "Kermit, let's go to the dance tonight!" as you model the conversation between the two puppets. Within-role suggestions might include, for example, "Andy, can you show Miss Piggy how Kermit can dance?" or "Let's dress the animals for the fancy party!"

Third, the use of the strategy of play materials in solitary play is based on the child's interest and past experiences. Introduction of familiar play materials is recommended for younger or new solitary players. Representational toys such as toy cars, dolls, and buildings are best at first; non-representational toys such as wood pieces, and fabric scraps are used by the more mature solitary player. Boundaries, the fourth strategy for the solitary player, are individual and very personal. Cries of "You can't play with me!" are common with the solitary playing child. The child's attention becomes focused on himself and the play theme to the exclusion of all others. The adult's job is to make these boundaries more permeable, flexible and less static by providing avenues for other children to enter into the world of the solitary player. For example, by commenting to the solitary player that, "Candy has a truck that could help you dig up the sand with your steam shovel!", your complimentary statements regard the boundaries of solitary play but yet soften them enough to permit another to play.

In using the fifth strategy, roles played, solitary-playing youngsters are free to choose their own character roles. The adult may suggest minor theme variations following those of the onlooker. Occasional use of modeling and within-play roles again helps to sustain and expand the youngster's interest. Role identity, consequent language growth, and a greater understanding of characterization and uses of objects result from the solitary players personalized choice of roles.

Parallel Play

With the strategy of time and space, young children benefit from playing near each other. Because play themes and objects change rapidly, and often without warning for parallel players, you should expect that time periods will be used creatively, actively and in a variety of ways. Providing open space which allows the youngsters, for instance, to march in a one-man band, as well as a small private space for block building are equally important for parallel play. As they parallel play, they will be within hearing and seeing range of one another. These time and space strategies provide for the assimilation of new themes and ideas. The second strategy, guidance, is necessary for parallel play. In using the strategy in parallel play, the adult's commenting occasionally about the play of each child encourages and reinforces play patterns. For example, three year old Heidi grabs the stuffed giraffe and scolds, "You've been naughty, Jeremy! Now, you must go the bed without any chocolate cake!" Four year old Alonzo, holding a stuffed unicorn, is soon overheard saying, "Jeremy giraffe is in bed! He was naughty at dinner time!" At this point, you can remark to both youngsters, "Maybe Jeremy and the unicorn can play blocks tomorrow!" By introducing new ideas indirectly, you guide them to extend and discover patterns and sequences in their own play. In addition, the children, hear and observe novel uses of familar objects, resulting in vocabulary, language and creativity advances.

In parallel play, representational toys, which maximize the play materials category — dress-up clothing, dolls and vehicle toys — are ideal. These toys quickly spark imagination of the parallel players because they have functional uses which can be easily modeled. Whenever possible, purchasing at least two similar or identical sets of each toy assists children in the development of parallel play. Children in parallel play can use the same type of object which contributes to their play as their needs arise. Boundaries, the fourth strategy for parallel play, are more flexible than those of solitary play. Parallel players do interact freely with one another. And, even though they more commonly interact "at one another," they move independently in and out of these routines. The "roles played" strategy in parallel play proceeds best when the adult follows the child's lead in player assignments. Children of similar interests and ages can facilitate each other's parallel play and role assignments.

Associative and Cooperative Play

Both in the center and home you can establish a background rich in opportunities for dramatic and sociodramatic play. Dramatic and sociodramatic play involves elements of both make-believe and imitation. Adult explanations, direct guidance and cooperation assume larger roles in these than with the other types of social play. For example, compared with other play stages, you can, in associative and cooperative play: (a) explain your reasons for actions; (b) break down complex actions into simple units of action; (c) answer child's questions concerning play choices; and (d) directly guide and model desirable play patterns. Additionally, describing wishes, future and past events and reading and discussing stories with the child are additional tools of dramatic and sociodramatic play. In using the first intervention the strategy of time and space, special places and times allotted for play welcome the children to play situations. Time and space set the stage for actions as well. The amount of time and space used in associative and cooperative play increases as compared with other types of play. These greater amounts of space and time are needed for children to use a variety of play actions, try out novel activities and go into greater depth and more detailed elaboration of their play.

Adult guidance, the second intervention strategy, provides for enhancing child's play and his repertoire of play actions. For example, encouraging positive social relationships will favorably influence the child's cooperation with peers in play. Guiding the child to play with different children and reinforcing the positive behaviors increases the child's social readiness and ability. Your verbal comments encourage the child to handle the objects imitatively during the playtime. Dramatic and sociodramatic play are stimulated by using suggestions, such as, "See the cars, trains, and buildings! Perhaps you and Heather could play 'big city' with them!" and "Look at the pretty new doll! Go and see if Elizabeth and Adam will help you to rock and feed her!" Speech, the central tool in dramatic and sociodramatic play, becomes a handy substitute for elements which the child wishes to include in the play. Through guidance using modeling, the adult enhances and stimulates the child's role-taking ability. For example, you might say, "Peter, let's pretend that the table is a bus. We'll crawl underneath it and take a trip to the dairy farm!" With these suggestions, the props and scenery become alive and are real to the players. The adult communicates enthusiasm and acceptance both verbally and nonverbally throughout the sequence. Using the strategies of nodding, exciting clapping, stooping to the children's level, interjecting comments, questions, and suggestions, and acting as a play episode participant, the adult joins in the fun.

The third strategy is play materials. In order for children to engage in dramatic and sociodramatic play they need varied toys and play materials. For example, cardboard squares, foil stars, empty paper towel rolls, empty shoe boxes, and crayons can all be used by youngsters in their sociodramatic play. With these materials, Philip, Sonya, Nancy, Carrie, and John, for example, begin to play "mailman!" They say, "Who will be our mail carrier? We'll need a dog that barks!" They plan the roles and use the materials and carry out the enactments of the "mailman." Each child interacts, converses, and moves according to roles. Body contact with other sociodramatic players as well as physical arrangement of the props and objects enables them to nonverbally communicate. Resultant social growth, language development and event sequencing are the rewards of using varied play materials in dramatic and sociodramatic play.

Boundaries in dramatic and sociodramatic play begin to change and are more flexible than at other stages of play. Rather than constructing barriers between themselves and their play, the children welcome involvement and participation from other youngsters. By merely suggesting that they want to play in a sociodramatic play episode, additional youngsters are included for the contributions that they can make to the group.

In using the strategy of roles in dramatic and sociodramatic play, the youngster includes great detail. As the children elaborate and completely describe the characters, they make their dramatic and sociodramatic play routines lively. With play at this level, the youngsters can rotate roles and enact the same episode over and over again. With each enactment of the same episode, the roles, play materials, and outcomes of the play episode differ markedly. Role changes coincide with, and facilitate, the youngsters developmental needs and interests.

In sum, whether children are playing in onlooker, solitary, and parallel fashion or whether the play is associative or cooperative, your role in the play is paramount. The adult in the center or the home is truly one of the child's most influential play and learning motivators. A role, so filled with potential, must not be considered lightly.

REFERENCES

Axline, V. M. *Play therapy*. New York: Ballantine Books, 1947.

Curry, N., and Arnaud, S. Cognitive implications in the children's spontaneous role play. *Theory into Practice*, 1974, *13*, 273-277.

Parten, M. Social participation among preschool children. *Journal of Abnormal Psychology*, 1932, *27*, 243-269.

Pellegrini, A. D., and Greene, H. Use of sequence-questioning paradigm to facilitate associative fluency in preschoolers. *Journal of Applied Developmental Psychology*, 1980, *1*, 189-200.

Piaget, J. *Play, dreams and imitation in childhood*. New York: W. W. Norton, 1962.

Singer, J. (Ed.). *The child's world of make-believe: Experimental studies of children's play*. New York: Academic Press, 1973.

Smilansky, S. *The effects of sociodramatic play on disadvantaged preschool children*. New York: Wiley, 1968.

Yawkey, T. D., and Fox, F. D. Evaluative intervention research in child's play. *The Journal of Research and Development in Education*, 1981, *14* (3), 40-57.

COMMUNITY SERVICES: AN ANALYSIS OF REFERRALS

Marilyn Mennis, MSW

ABSTRACT. Making successful referrals to community agencies is a complex and difficult process. It requires professional expertise, cooperative relationships between agencies and mandates which foster referrals. This paper will examine referral issues from the perspective of the service level agency to agency interrelationships as well as the systemic impediments to referrals found in legal mandates, funding, and confidentiality requirements.

The puzzling child is often a child who requires intervention in more than one service system. All children are "served" by the educational system and to some degree by the health system. For the child with a problem there are a multiplicity of community agencies, any one or more of which may need to be involved. Such community agencies include mental health, mental retardation, family services, child welfare, corrections, drug and alcohol, protective services, and more. Thus interagency relationships are a fact of life for any human service agency which serves children and families.

Over the past 15-20 years there has been a proliferation of laws and court decisions at the federal and state levels mandating a variety of services to children. Unfortunately, this proliferation of services mandated and funded by government has not addressed the problem of services to children who need more than one type of intervention. A Task Force examining mental health services for children in Penn-

---

Marilyn Mennis is Director of Program Development, Child Psychiatry Center, at St. Christopher's Hospital for Children, 2603 North 5th Street, Philadelphia, PA 19133.

sylvania reported that children with multiple diagnoses and handicaps are chronically underserved due to the inability of systems oriented to a single problem to provide cooperative services.[1]

The problem is typically attributed to a lack of coordination between agencies or helping professionals;[2] and a new service concept has evolved to accommodate the problem thus define—case management, unified systems of intake and referral, and umbrella human service agencies at the local level. Some of the problems in referrals are amenable to solution through improved interagency coordination.

What these solutions do not address, however, are the systemic problems which impede cooperative and coordinated relationships, e.g., conflicting and contradictory mandates, exclusionary funding streams, confidentiality requirements, and questions of which agency or system is responsible in particular instances and which is obligated to fund the service (often requiring a determination of which problem or diagnosis is "primary"). Scarce funding exacerbates the situation since the multi-problem child is often an expensive child to serve. This set of problems is not readily amenable to solution at the local service agency level but rather requires the cooperation of state agency officials and a willingness to write program requirements in concert with one another.

Some states have attempted to address such systemic problems through a comprehensive service approach. In 1972 Massachusetts passed a law mandating a comprehensive program of diagnosis and services to children with special needs.[3] In Pennsylvania, recognizing these systems problems, the General Assembly established in 1979 a Task Force on Exceptional Children[4] to examine the relationships and overlapping responsibilities between the major systems of care for exceptional children and to make recommendations.

What follows is an attempt to examine referral and coordination relationships between child serving agencies which affect a family's ability to obtain needed services for their child.

What Are Referrals and Are They Successful?

"A referral is a professional service in assisting an individual...to avail himself or herself of the appropriate community social resource or service when the request for help is beyond the [professional's] function or training."[5] It may be with the expectation that the new relationship will supplant the old[6] or that it will supplement the existing service.

To move between services is a difficult process for a client. New intakes, locations, rules and eligibility requirements act as impediments to service and result in a high rate of attrition.[7] Such impediments may be even more critical with respect to children, for whom consistency and continuity are essential components of a successful intervention. As a result, as studies have shown, many clients never follow through on referrals and the attrition rate following the initial visit is high.[6,8]

Equally important as the question "are referrals successful?" is the question "do referrals occur?"; that is, are the gatekeepers willing to make referrals. Most, if not all, of the organized human service systems include a referral component as an integral service. While they do not always work at optimal effectiveness, there is a basic assumption that referrals are important. This is less true of the medical profession, and because physicians are primary gatekeepers in our society, this is a critical lack, especially for children. Efforts to train pediatricians in mental health issues, for example, have been less than successful[9] and even when they are aware of community mental health, doctors tend not to refer their patients,[10] particularly to the publicly funded agencies. Since physicians tend to establish referral relationships with other individual practitioners rather than with facilities (except of course for hospitals), one approach might be for individual professionals in community agencies to develop relationships with local physicians. It would seem essential that we convince one of the primary gatekeepers for children that community services are an important, credible and legitimate resource for the puzzling child.

Components of the (Successful) Referral

Most agencies serving children are oriented toward referrals. It is often built into the mandating law or regulations — case management, service brokering, unified intake and referral are common concepts. Even given this orientation, problems obviously exist as evidenced by the failure rates cited above. Faulty referrals frustrate the client's effort to find help. They also frustrate the receiving agency and erode the relationship between referring and receiving agency.

The critical components of a referral are mechanics (how), appropriateness (why, to whom and when), expectations, and coordination.[6,11]

How to Refer

Several studies have shown that the way in which a referral is made will determine its success or failure. "Active" referrals in which the referring agency makes the contact are more successful than passive referrals in which the client is told where to go and left to his/her own resources.[8] The referring agent must work on the client's motivation and confidence in the new agency, and help the client work through potential feelings of rejection from the referring agency and professional.[6] In this regard, the maintenance of the original relationship, particularly for children, may assist in the transition to a new service and increase the chances for the success of the referral.

From the agency perspective, referrals must follow procedures established by the receiving agency. Relationships between agencies often break down simply as a result of not complying with such procedures. Since each agency has its own intake process, it may be difficult for referring agents to learn every other agency's procedures. Uniform referral and intake procedures between frequently used agencies help to resolve these problems.

Appropriateness of and Expectations for the Referral

An appropriate referral is one which is made for the right reasons, at the right time and to the right agency. Expectations as to what the referral will accomplish for the client must be realistic.

In a study of interagency relationships among children's agencies in a suburban county (Chester) near Philadelphia,[11] *several problems in the area of appropriateness surfaced. The timing of referrals was often cited as a problem in that they frequently occur at times of crisis rather than early enough to avert the crisis. A second important element in an appropriate referral is knowing which service to request. The mental health agencies in the Chester County study chafed under what they considered to be inappropriate referrals for psychiatric evaluations when in their assessment such referrals often required psychological testing instead. At the same time, the referring agencies were upset that their requests were being re-evaluated by the receiving

---

*Supported by the Pennsylvania Department of Public Welfare, Office of Mental Health. Project directors M. Mennis and J. Noone.

agency. Both the question of timing and the nature of the request can be resolved by discussions between the agencies involved, though such attempts have not always been successful.

Expectations about what a referral can accomplish may affect the outcome of the referral, particularly when those expectations are conveyed to the client. Unrealistic expectations, however, also lead to poor inter-agency relationships which ultimately affects referral interactions. In the Chester County study it was found that expectations for what an adequate amount of mental health services can accomplish run high and far exceed what even a full complement of services could do. One response suggested that "the MH/MR system is underfunded and understaffed causing emotional health of families to further deteriorate....If psychiatric treatment were more readily available to dysfunctional adults, children's problems would be considerably alleviated."[11] Such an analysis reflects a degree of expectation which the mental health system, even with adequate resources, could never meet. It also reflects the incredible and legitimate frustration felt by professionals working with problem-ridden families. Finally it underscores the expectations for services created by government mandates which inadequate funding does not permit agencies to meet.

Mental health agencies are caught in expectations not only of the "curative" capability of mental health treatment but also of their ability to make valid and reliable predictions about future behavior (e.g., in probation, custody and abuse situations). Mental health professionals understandably feel that they are expected to perform miracles. Educational professionals similarly feel that they are expected to be all things to all children. Such a situation does not provide an environment in which positive referral relationships can exist. Agencies need to clearly establish the limits of their capability and communicate these limits to referring agencies.

Accurate knowledge about community resources is therefore a critical component in appropriateness of referrals and in delimiting frustration resulting from unrealistic expectations. Resource directories may be a partial solution to this problem.[12] However, such directories often do not describe the nature of the services, eligibility and service limitations in sufficient detail, if at all. It is, therefore, necessary for agencies which make relatively more frequent use of one another's services to clarify for each other what can and cannot be provided, in what time frame and to whom. Surprisingly, this apparently obvious solution is not often used.

Interagency Coordination and Collaboration on Referred Cases

While some referrals are intended to supplant one service with another, many referrals are intended to supplement existing services. For a child, any service is in addition to their participation in a school setting. Thus for children's services, coordination is of critical concern to avoid contradictory and conflicting treatment and advice. The lack of coordinated activity on behalf of a child or family can increase the chances of family disintegration.[2]

While it is difficult to know how many children are being served simultaneously by more than one agency (with the exception of school), those cases actively known to two or more agencies tend to require a disproportionate amount of time, as they are frequently multiproblem families, often in crisis and very demanding of the service systems.[11]

Information-sharing is critical. When the referring agency is continuing to serve the child, feedback and follow-up should be provided by the receiving agency as to goals, objectives and services being provided, with periodic reports as to progress.

Equally important is collaboration on the development of goals, objectives and interventions between involved agencies. Without exception, the agencies which participated in the Chester County study identified this as an area which needed improvement. While the school and the agency or the two agencies may coincidentally follow parallel and consistent paths in providing services to a child, they may be equally likely to develop quite different and contradictory approaches, resulting in the failure of one or both treatment approaches.

Interagency coordination and collaboration are not easy to accomplish. Confidentiality requirements impede inter-professional communications on individual cases. Constraints on staff time make it difficult to hold interagency case conferences. Professionals may feel threatened by the intervention of other professionals with different approaches. The service environment in one setting may not be amenable to changes suggested by a newly involved professional (e.g., a teacher may not be able to alter the classroom structure, or the child welfare agency change a placement or remove a child from home). It is incumbant on agencies, nonetheless, to attempt to work together if the child or family is to be helped.

One approach which has been found helpful in referral and

collaboration relationships is the *liaison model*. Again, in Chester County, in every situation where a formal liaison person was identified in one agency to link with another, the relationship between agencies improved. Where a formal liaison relationship ceased to exist (usually because of funding), the linkage deteriorated. The existence of the liaison person seems to impact not only on information sharing, collaboration and problem solving, but also on the number of referrals generated.[11]

While it is obviously not possible to cover the field with liaison workers for every agency to every other agency, the success with this type of formal relationship is suggestive. Perhaps in those instances where frequent interactions occur, or where problems between service systems or agencies have been identified, a formal liaison would be desirable.

Systems Problems Affecting Referrals

Many of the problems identified in completing referrals for community services are amenable to correction by the professionals and agencies who make and receive referrals. There remains, however, a set of problems which cannot be resolved at the local level, and which unfortunately cause enormous frustration for service providers and clients alike.

Contradictory Mandates and Funding Exclusions

Each service system has its own laws, regulations and funding requirements. Laws mandating services in each system tend to mandate in isolation. They assume that a child has only one, or at least a primary, problem which defines them into or out of a particular service system. When they do make reference to other services, it is often to exclude funding (e.g., child welfare cannot pay for residential placement in a mental health facility); or there is a lack of clarity as to who is responsible for what (e.g., "related services" under PL 94-142, the Education for All Handicapped Children Act).

What lawmakers often do not recognize is that a series of such laws creates overlapping jurisdictions with no designation of primary responsibility for a multi-problem child and no ability to share funding resources on behalf of a particular child. Since each funding stream wants to be the last dollar in, and often excludes anything which could conceivably be paid for by another system, a child with multiple problems has much difficulty obtaining service in any system. When funding is tight and reimbursements are restricted, any given system interprets responsibility as belonging to any other system. Thus, for example, a child who is mentally ill and also dependent and neglected and is in need of residential service is often shunted back and forth between child welfare and mental health. In another frequently discussed example, is education obligated to provide and/or pay for "related services" under PL 94-142 (e.g., psychotherapy or intermittent catheterization) or does the other system (mental health or health) assume the responsibility and the cost?[13,14] Responsibility for residential services provided in concert with the educational program is an equally knotty question with at least three service systems as well as various advocacy groups in conflict over who is obligated to pay. The courts have often been called upon to resolve some of these jurisdictional disputes.

Further complicating the situation is the fact that some services require that clients be charged fees while others, notably special education, require that no financial liability be imposed. If a service such as psychotherapy is considered a "related service" and included in the child's educational plan, and the child is referred to a mental health clinic where client fees are mandated, there is an inevitable conflict. The laws are not clear as to who pays — the school system, the mental health system, or the parents.

Finally, agencies which pay for services usually want some measure of control over the nature of the service provided.[14] Shared funding on behalf of a client is therefore even more difficult to achieve.

While in principle these various funding streams could be mixed on behalf of a particular child, the lack of a mandate to do so from the state authorities, limited financial resources in each system, difficulties in determining who has primary responsibility, issues of control, and varied requirements for client payment of fees make it difficult to do so. Such mixing could be accomplished by extending to agencies the ability to contribute to or to purchase services from another system, or to jointly develop and fund a service, or by licensing agencies in more than one system when they are related. For example, child welfare could be permitted to pay for the non-treatment residential costs in a mental health facility for a child eligible for its services. All of these approaches currently exist; however, they exist in spite of the mandates and are fraught with difficulties in meeting the requirements and exclusions of all of their licensing and funding authorities.

Confidentiality

Confidentiality and client access to records is another set of public mandates which creates a systemic impediment to interagency cooperation and collaboration on individual referrals. While it would be difficult to oppose the protections which have been developed with respect to access to and distribution of patient/client records, it must be recognized that exchange of information essential to case collaboration and once common among professionals, is now inhibited by numerous mechanical constraints.[15] Not only do these cumbersome procedures inhibit information sharing, and therefore coordinated intervention, in some cases they also inhibit the referrals themselves. Because laws, such as the one in Illinois, make no provision for disclosure in situations in which the use might serve a good purpose, professionals are left in a quandary. For example, such restrictions may block a child protective service unit from making a referral on an unproven case to a social service agency or even to a unit within their own agency.[15] Since some interpretations of confidentiality extend to the "fact" that a client is receiving a service, feedback to a referral source is also thwarted.

Access to records by clients presents an additional problem area affecting exchange of information among professionals and service providers. The Family Educational Rights and Privacy Act of 1974, known as the Buckley Amendment, gives parents and children access to the child's school records. Reports sent by other agencies such as mental health centers to the schools are in a grey area as to whether they are part of the school record and therefore accessible or are protected as belonging to the originator of the report and not the school. The possibility that such reports will be released makes mental health and other professionals very wary about sending reports and has widened the communications gap between mental health centers and the schools.[16]

Some of the difficulties with confidentiality between involved agencies are resolvable. Providing information on each agency's confidentiality mandates will clarify and define the imposed limits and reduce unrealistic expectations for information-sharing. Agencies could develop inter-agency policies and routine procedures for obtaining consent for release of information. They can attempt to define for themselves where the grey areas are and agree on interpretations which they will all follow.

Yet it is important that lawmakers and government officials begin to work together to develop policies which reduce these constraints without, of course, abridging the protections for which they were designed.

Conclusion

Referral relationships involve complicated and complex interactions. The success or failure of referrals and the ability of agencies to respond to referrals is dependent on many factors. While certainly not perfect, the major children's service systems have developed a degree of sophistication in coordination on behalf of their clients. Additional work can be done in the areas of training in how to refer, the use of liaison workers, the development of uniform referral procedures and case coordination mechanisms, and the development of more comprehensive resource directories. However, we have now just begun to recognize and address the broader and non-agency-specific impediments to referrals. Fragmentation of services at the local level is perhaps no longer the problem. Fragmentation of program mandates, policies and funding, often developed in isolation from one another, is the real culprit. Inter-agency or inter-departmental agreements at the State and Federal level is essential to the resolution of these newly defined problems.

REFERENCES

1. Department of Public Welfare, Commonwealth of Pennsylvania Mental Health Services for the Children and Youth of Pennsylvania. Final Report of the Task Force on Mental Health Planning for Children and Youth. April 13, 1979.

2. Selig, A. L. The myth of the multi-problem family. *American Journal of Orthopsychiatry*, 1976, *46*, 526-532.

3. England, M. J. Children's services in Massachusetts: "...and the first will come last." *American Journal of Orthopsychiatry*, 1980, *50*, 205-210.

4. Commonwealth of Pennsylvania. Senate Resolution No. 202. June 27, 1979.

5. Millard, T. L. School counseling and referral. *Journal of the International Association of Pupil Personnel Workers*, 1977, *21*, 112-116.

6. Cary, A. R., Black, K. J., Neider, G. G. Upping the odds on the referral gamble. *School Counsel*, 1978, *25*, 186-190.

7. Daniels, R. S. Changing human delivery systems: Their influence on psychiatric training. *American Journal of Psychiatry*, 1973, *130*, 1232-1236.

8. Sudak, H. S., Sawyer, J. B., Spring, G. K., et al. High Referral success rates in a crisis center. *Hospital and Community Psychiatry*, 1977, *28*, 530-532.

9. Child Psychiatry Center at St. Christopher's Hospital for Children. Interdisciplinary Continuing Education Project in Child and Family Mental Health. NIMH Grant # 1 T 15 MH 15435-01, 1978-1981.

10. Perkins, D. V., Thompson, J. R. An assessment of physicians' attitudes toward community mental health. *Community Mental Health Journal*, 1974, *10*, 282-291.

11. Child Psychiatry Center at St. Christopher's Hospital for Children. Mental Health Services to Children and Families. Final Report. April 1979.

12. Tippett, J., Owens, R., and Frome, F. Indirect services and referral system for community mental health centers: Implementation and methods of measurement. *Community Mental Health Journal*, 1974, *10*, 450-465.

13. Bryan, E. Administrative concerns and schools' relationship with private practicing physicians. *Journal of School Health*, 1979, *49*, 157-163.

14. Scanlon, R. G. Testimony on Education for All Handicapped Children Act (PL 94-142). Before U.S. Senate Subcommittee on the Handicapped. October 3, 1979.

15. Foster, L. M. State confidentiality laws: The Illinois act as model for new legislation in other states. *American Journal of Orthopsychiatry*, 1980, *50*, 659-665.

16. Drake, E. A., and Barden, J. I. Confidentiality and interagency communication: Effect of the Buckley amendment. *Hospital and Community Psychiatry*, 1978, *29*, 312-315.

ETHICAL ISSUES ASSOCIATED WITH THE IMPLEMENTATION OF PL 94-142: IMPLICATIONS FOR THE NEXT DECADE

Cheryl L. Kinsey, MA
Patricia A. Morrissey, PhD

ABSTRACT. This article describes the intent of PL 94-142, The Education for All Handicapped Children Act of 1975. This law requires that each handicapped child has available to him or her a free appropriate public education. The law also requires that certain procedures be followed in the provision of such an education. The article also outlines four ethical conflicts which emerge as local systems implement the law and it suggests how they may be resolved. We emphasize the importance of parent and school cooperation, particularly in this time of federal, state, and local cuts in education budgets.

Introduction

With the passage of PL 94-142, The Education for All Handicapped Children Act, Congress guaranteed a free, appropriate public education to all handicapped children between the ages of 3 and 21 by 1978. The intent of this law was to correct wide-spread injustices in educational programming for disabled children and provide them with

Cheryl L. Kinsey is on the Professional Staff of the Select Education Subcommittee, Committee on Education and Labor, U.S. House of Representatives and Patricia A. Morrissey is a Minority Legislative Associate, Committee on Education and Labor, U.S. House of Representatives, Washington, D.C. 20515.

the learning opportunities they needed to become self-sufficient, productive members of society.

Prior to the enactment of this law, it was estimated that half of the nation's 8 million handicapped were being denied an appropriate education and as many as one million children were totally excluded from school.[1] This new legislation went further than any other law in our history to try and reach these children and change the direction of their lives.

The intent of PL 94-142 is stated simply: "to assure that all handicapped children have available to them...a free and appropriate education which emphasizes special education and related services to meet their unique needs."[2] Under the law the federal government becomes a partner with the states and agrees to assist them in fulfilling their obligation to handicapped children (Riley, Nash, and Hunt, 1978). However, in order to qualify for this assistance states must submit a plan detailing how they will carry out this commitment to the goal of free and appropriate education for all handicapped children. Much of these funds "flow-through" to the local education agencies provided that certain requirements of the Act are met. In order to obtain this money, they must submit plans to the state outlining how they will comply with the provisions of the law at the local level.[3]

Through these very specific provisions of PL 94-142, the federal government has provided the states with a process for enabling them to guard against possible lawsuits for failure to adequately address the needs of handicapped children (Council of School Attorneys, 1980). If states choose not to receive federal assistance under PL 94-142, however, this does not relieve them of their responsibility to provide appropriate programs for disabled children under Section 504 of the Rehabilitation Act of 1973 (National Association of State Directors of Special Education and the National Association of State Boards of Education, 1979). The intent of PL 94-142 is that specific administrative procedures be put into place to ensure *all* handicapped children the appropriate educational opportunities that are available to their non-handicapped peers.

In this article we will review the principle provisions of PL 94-142 as they relate to "treatment"—those that guarantee a free appropriate public education. Given that framework we will address selected ethical issues that arise in the application of PL 94-142 to individual cases as well as strategies for increasing the possibility of doing what is right—the ethical response. This is a time of uncertainty regarding the future of the federal role in education. Although PL 94-142 offers specificity in protection and services, we must be prepared for the possible alteration or "repeal" of the law. As of May, 1982, the administration had not formally submitted to the Congress a bill to amend the Education for All Handicapped Children Act. From the Department of Education position, the proposed amendments provide state and local education agencies more flexibility while protecting the concept of free appropriate public education. However, draft documents would seem to eliminate IEP as we know it and weaken some due process procedures.

Major Provisions

The basic principle underlying PL 94-142 is that *all* handicapped children must be afforded the opportunity for appropriate educational services. Therefore, all school systems are obligated to establish a system to locate all children with disabilities.[4] If a parent consents to an evaluation for a child suspected of having a disability, a battery of racially and culturally non-discriminatory and language-appropriate tests will be given by an interdisciplinary team of professionals. The results of this evaluation, along with other informally-collected data, will be used to determine eligibility for special education and related services. In addition, it will be used to determine what kinds of approaches might be employed in setting up an education program for the child.

If a child is found eligible for special education and related services, PL 94-142 requires that an Individual Education Program (IEP)[5] be prepared in consultation with the parents, and if possible, the child. Other education personnel participating in this "staffing" should have knowledge of the testing battery used in the evaluation, the child and the resources of the school system. This document states the specific short and long term education goals and specific services to be provided for the individual child over one year. To assure that this program is being appropriately implemented, the IEP must be evaluated and updated annually in a meeting with the "staffing team." Once this IEP is agreed upon by both parents and teachers, the child's placement is not to be changed unless it is agreeable to all parties involved.

One of the basic considerations in designing appropriate education programs for handicapped children must be the strong emphasis in the law on educating children in the least restrictive environment.[6] This provision requires that to the maximum extent appropriate handicapped children must be educated with their non-handicapped peers. Only in cases where it is impossible to work out a satisfactory placement on these terms should a handicapped child be educated in a segregated school or class. Through this provision children who were formally educated in residential settings or special schools would be given the opportunity to be "mainstreamed" into the regular school setting.

Other protections provided by PL 94-142 are the assurance of due process[7] for both parents and school personnel and the assurance of confidentiality in the maintenance of records.[8] Any party may exercise their right to due process in procedures related to identification, evaluation and placement as well as appropriate educational programming. If this occurs, and an agreement cannot be reached through an administrative review at the local level, an impartial due process hearing may be requested. In order to assure that this procedure is handled efficiently and effectively, PL 94-142 has specific timelines within which each step in the process must be completed. If one of the parties is dissatisfied with the decision reached at the local level, the decision may be appealed to the state. If the state level review is unsatisfactory to one of the parties, it may request civil court action.

Parents of handicapped children are also offered protection under PL 94-142 by its provision for confidentiality in the maintenance of records. This safeguard requires that only the school personnel directly involved with the education program for a specific child are permitted to have access to his records, unless parent permission is received. All special education records must be kept in secure vaults and those allowed access to them must be documented.

Ethical Issues

While PL 94-142 has provided a great promise for assuring equity in services to all children, both non-handicapped and handicapped, many age-old problems have been slow to change. Educators, administrators, legislators and parents have debated the provisions of this law repeatedly in an effort to provide remedies to these problems that will be acceptable to all parties. Unfortunately, while PL 94-142 sets a tone and direction for schools to follow when dealing with handicapped children which increases the likelihood that they will receive a free, appropriate, public education, it does not guarantee that this will occur for every child.

In many cases a school system with limited resources, both in terms of funds and placement options, may be forced to make educational programming decisions based on these limitations. In other cases the school personnel making the critical decisions on appropriate placements may be governed by the wishes of higher level administrators who may dictate how placements are to be made (Education Turnkey Systems, Inc., 1978; National Education Association, 1978). Parents may be intimidated by the authority vested in a school administrator, and therefore not offer suggestions or register complaints. Administrators, on the other hand, may be concerned about the likelihood of a due process request and consequently not be open to a free exchange with parents. Teachers may be given the responsibility for writing draft and final IEPs, and yet not have influence over critical decisions such as placement or the timing, amount, and nature of related services. In such a context teachers may view their responsibilities related to writing IEPs more as clerical tasks than as professional obligations (Goldsmith et al., 1980; Yoshida et al., 1978).

Another ethical issue stemming from the implementation of PL 94-142 is labeling (Reschly and Lamprecht, 1978). While PL 94-142 does not encourage or discourage the use of labels such as mentally retarded, learning disabled or emotionally disturbed, it does require that a count of children in each disability category be taken and recorded for funding purposes. The law emphasizes an evaluation of each child's strengths and weaknesses with this information being specifically stated in the IEP, however, labeling provides a professional short-cut in communicating with other education personnel in addressing a child's specific needs. Although some school systems have chosen to provide non-categorical programs, the children are still perceived by those persons who work with them as in some way deviant from the norm. When PL 94-142 was first enacted it appeared that parents felt most threatened by the fact that their child would receive a label if he was placed in a special education program. Some research now suggests that many parents actually need labels to justify the existence of a problem. Consequently, children with handicaps are most often labeled and grouped by such labels.

In addition to these issues, the very specific procedures in the Act for due process have in some cases produced an adversarial relationship between parents and school personnel—countering the effectiveness of other procedures (Boston, 1977). Many times rather than developing an attitude that both parties were working together toward a common goal—it has appeared that one side was trying to "do the other in" losing sight of the needs of the child involved. The specificity of services required by PL 94-142 has made it easier for one side to find fault with the other.

Lastly, the confidentiality requirements of PL 94-142 may impede the development of a functional relationship between program planning and classroom practice. For example, in many schools IEPs are locked in the principal's office in observance of the requirements that personal records of children should be in a secure place, a place of controlled access. Such a policy may contribute to the development of the perception that IEPs are merely compliance documents which may or may not reflect classroom practice. Furthermore, if only some school personnel have ready access to student files, then others may believe that they are less responsible and accountable for what is contained in IEPs. Parents are sometimes confused with the security surrounding their children's records. This confusion may lead to a perception that there may be mysterious information in the records, and that school personnel are generally guarded about what they will share with parents. In cases where information must be shared among professionals, the failure of a parent to give permission for access to their child's records may actually provide a roadblock to the implementation of an appropriate education program for their children (Education Turnkey Systems, 1978).

In spite of the constraints we have outlined, the intent of the law may still be achieved if school systems seek to clarify the roles of all planning participants—administrators, teachers, and parents—before IEP meetings and if they endorse decision-making by consensus both when planning for individual children and when developing or selecting general school policies and procedures.

In the initial effort to implement PL 94-142 in 1978, school personnel did not have time to reflect on how best to respond to the many requirements of the law. Now is perhaps the time to reflect on current school practice and make changes to reduce unnecessary burdens on teachers, administrators and facilitate more parent involvement which should ultimately improve services to handicapped children. For example, prior to meetings participants should agree to some general role guidelines. Meetings may proceed more smoothly because participants have a common orientation about an appropriate division of responsibility. Such guidelines may include the recognition that: the administrator would assume the primary responsibility for explaining and making resource commitments (Frith, 1981); direct service personnel would offer instructional strategies and a rationale for using them; the parents would give their perception of the child's strengths, weaknesses and general needs; and the child, if present, would share his/her preferences and goals. If participants are willing to assume these roles and share information with each other, an integrated, comprehensive individualized plan is likely to result (Robson, 1981).

An important component of planning is the decision-making process. We feel that for decision-making to result in appropriate programming for a child or effective policies for a school system as a whole it would be decision-making by consensus. Such decision-making may be characterized in terms of: acceptance of diverse and overlapping expertise; the availability of real choices; no pre-ordained decisions; the provision of information in a timely manner; the drafting or selection of information which is comprehensible and relevant; the availability of rules for resolving differences; and the recognition of the fact that unresolved differences ultimately harm children by delaying effective services.

Although we have offered suggestions that may improve the school's response to the handicapped child under the current mandate—PL 94-142, we have also offered suggestions which may be even more applicable if the mandate were altered or repealed. For example, if Congress passes new legislation which gives local school systems increased discretion over the use of federal funds, parents will have an increased responsibility to try and influence decisions which affect resource allocations throughout the school system. If Congressional legislation reduces federal involvement in and assurance of due process, then resolution of conflicts dealing with the appropriateness of educational practice will have to be found within the local education community. If funding from the federal government is gradually but significantly reduced, parents must be willing to assist schools, at least to the same extent they place demands on schools. Coalitions of educators and parents that focus on improvements in the education system as a whole are likely to be more effective than narrowly-defined interest groups that pursue objectives that benefit a very few children.

Conclusion

In this article we have described the intent of PL 94-142, outlined four ethical issues which may emerge as local systems attempt to implement the law; suggested the value of role clarification and decision-making by consensus as indirect methods for improving services for handicapped children; and finally, proposed that the experience of parents and educators with PL 94-142 may be used to benefit all children in the 1980s. In order for our educational system to adapt to anticipated changes in federal education policy in the next decade, a strong partnership between parents and local educators must be formed. Adversarial relationships then may be set aside; the distinction between general and special education may be reduced; preferential treatment of some children may be stopped—because there will be a collective commitment to and understanding of the individual needs and rights of all children.

NOTES

1. The Education for All Handicapped Children Act of 1975. PL 94-142. U.S. Code: 20 U.S.C. 1411. C.F.D.A.: 13.499.
2. The Education for All Handicapped Children Act of 1975. PL 94-142. U.S. Code: 20 U.S.C. 1411. C.F.D.A.: 13.499.
3. *Federal Register*, August 23, 1977, Education of Handicapped Children. Implementation of Part B of the Education of the Handicapped Act. Subpart B.
4. *Federal Register*, August 23, 1977, Education of Handicapped Children. Implementation of Part B of the Education of the Handicapped Act. Subpart B, 121a.128; Subpart E, 1212a.530-121a.534.
5. *Federal Register*, August 23, 1977, Education of Handicapped Children. Implementation of Part B of the Education of the Handicapped Act. Subpart C, 121a.340-1212a.349.
6. *Federal Register*, August 23, 1977, Education of Handicapped Children. Implementation of Part B of the Education of the Handicapped Act. Subpart E, 121a.550-121a.556.
7. *Federal Register*, August 23, 1977, Education of Handicapped Children. Implementation of Part B of the Education of the Handicapped Act. Subpart E, 121a.500-121a.514.
8. *Federal Register*, August 23, 1977, Education of Handicapped Children. Implementation of Part B of the Education of the Handicapped Act. Subpart E, 1212a550-1212a.556.

REFERENCES

Boston, B. O. *Education policy and the education of all handicapped children act* (PL 94-142). Washington, D.C.: Institute for Educational Leadership.

Council of School Attorneys, National School Boards Association. *Schools and the law of the handicapped*. Washington, D.C., 1980.

Education Turnkey Systems, Inc. *Case study of the implementation of PL 94-142*. Washington, D.C., 1978.

Frith, G. H. "Advocate" vs. "professional employee". A question of priorities for special educators. *Exceptional Children*, 1981, *47*(7), 486-492.

Goldsmith, S., Strickland, B., Turnbull, A. P., & Curry, L. An observational analysis of the IEP Conference. *Exceptional Children*, 1980, *46*(4), 278-286.

National Association of State Directors of Special Education and the National Association of State Boards of Education. *Answering your questions about PL 94-142 and Section 504: A resource handbook*. Washington, D.C., 1979.

National Education Association. *A study report: Education of handicapped children: Consensus, conflict, and challenge*. Washington, D.C., 1978.

Reschly, D. J., & Lamprecht, M. R. Expectancy effects of labels: Factor of artifact. *Exceptional Children*, 1978, *46*(1), 55-58.

Riley, D. P., Nash, H. D., & Hunt, J. T. *National incentives in special education*. National Association of State Directors of Special Education, Washington, D.C., 1978.

Robson, D. L. Administering educational services for the handicapped: Role expectations and perceptions. *Exceptional Children*, 1981, *47*(5), 377-378.

Yoshida, R., Fenton, K., Kaufman, J. J., & Maxwell, J. P. Parental in special education pupil planning process: The school's perspective. *Exceptional Children*, 1978, *44*, 531-533.